COLOUR GUIDE

PICTURE TESTS

Neonatology And Paediatrics

Warren Hyer MB ChB MRCP
Senior Paediatric Registrar,
Northwick Park Hospital,
London

Roslyn Thomas MB BS FRCP
Consultant Paediatrician,
Northwick Park Hospital,
London

David Harvey MB FRCP DCH
Professor of Paediatrics and Neonatal Medicine,
Royal Postgraduate Medical School,
London

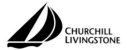

CHURCHILL
LIVINGSTONE

EDINBURGH LONDON MADRID MELBOURNE NEW YORK SAN FRANCISCO AND
TOKYO 1998

CHURCHILL LIVINGSTONE
Medical Division of Pearson Professional Limited

Distributed in the United States of America by Churchill
Livingstone Inc., 650 Avenue of the Americas, New York,
N.Y. 10011, and by associated companies, branches and
representatives throughout the world.

First Edition 1998

ISBN 0443 04956 4

British Library Cataloguing in Publication Data
A catalogue record for this book is available from the British
Library.

Library of Congress Cataloging in Publication Data
A catalog record for this book is available from the Library of
Congress.

Medical knowledge is constantly changing. As new
information becomes available, changes in treatment,
procedures, equipment and the use of drugs become
necessary. The authors and the publishers have, as far as it is
possible, taken care to ensure that the information given in
this text is accurate and up to date. However, readers are
strongly advised to confirm that the information, especially
with regard to drug usage, complies with current legislation
and standards of practice.

For Churchill Livingstone
Publisher
Timothy Horne

Project manager
Ninette Premdas

Project editor
Jim Killgore

Design
Erik Bigland

Project controller
Kay Hunston

The
publisher's
policy is to use
**paper manufactured
from sustainable forests**

Produced by Longman Asia Limited, Hong Kong
SWTC/01

Preface

This book is for whiling away the long hours in the middle of the night when you have nothing else to do but test your knowledge. We hope that it will be suitable for undergraduate medical students, paediatric nurses and paediatricians at all stages of their careers, especially those taking examinations.

London   W. H.

1998   R. T.

                                                                              D. H.

Acknowledgements

Drs Robert Feldman, Irene Roberts, Francis Cowan and Professor John Walker Smith who provided some of the photographs and scans.

Contents

Questions

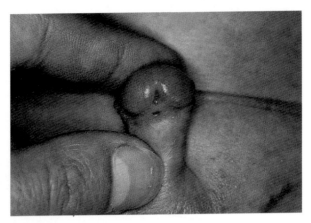

1. **This is the penis of a newborn infant.**

a. What is the diagnosis?
b. What are the associated findings?
c. How is this treated?

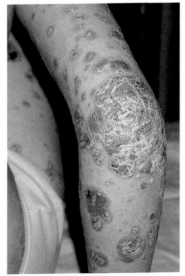

2. **This rash has been present for 5 months.**

a. What is the diagnosis?
b. What are the associated findings?
c. What is the treatment?

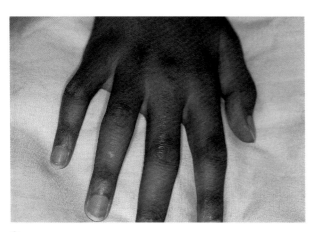

3. This 8-year-old girl presented with a painful hand, rash and splenomegaly.

a. What is the differential diagnosis?
b. What are the associated findings?
c. What is the treatment?

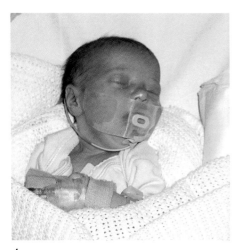

4. This is a 1-day-old infant.

a. What is the diagnosis?
b. Describe any associated findings.
c. What is the management?

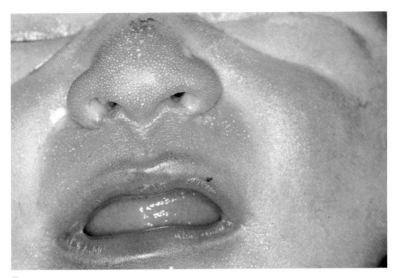

5. White spots on the nose of a newborn.

a. What is the diagnosis?
b. What is the treatment?

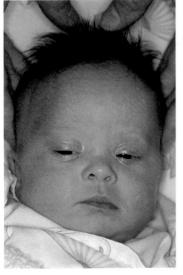

6.

a. What is the diagnosis?
b. How could this be determined antenatally?
c. What are the gastrointestinal manifestations?

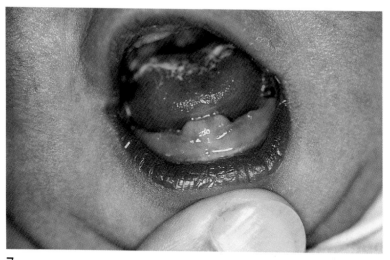

7. Alveolar margin of a newborn infant.

a. What is the diagnosis?
b. What are the complications?

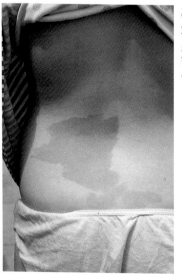

8. This 4-year-old girl has bone pain and gynaecomastia.

a. What is the diagnosis?
b. What are the associated findings?
c. What is the differential diagnosis of the skin lesion?

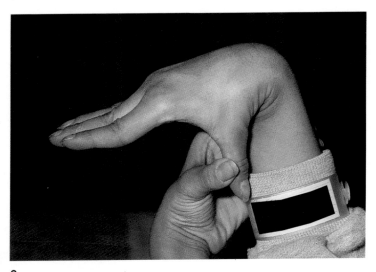

9.

a. What is the diagnosis?
b. What are the other features?
c. What is the treatment?

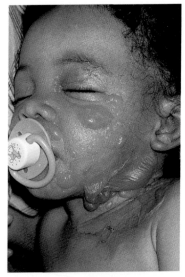

10.

a. What is the diagnosis?
b. How would one assess the child?
c. How would one treat?

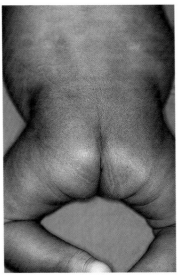

11. This 1-month-old infant was referred with suspected non-accidental injury.

a. What is the diagnosis?
b. What is the treatment?

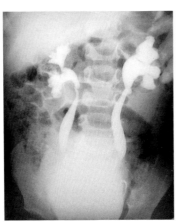

12. This X-ray is of a 2-year-old girl with recurrent urinary tract infections.

a. What is the diagnosis?
b. What other radiological investigations are indicated?
c. What is the management?

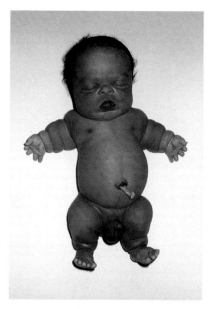

A

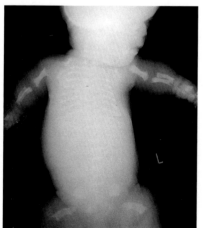

B

13. **This photograph and X-ray are of a newborn baby who died 1 hour after birth.**

a. What is the diagnosis?
b. What is the inheritance?

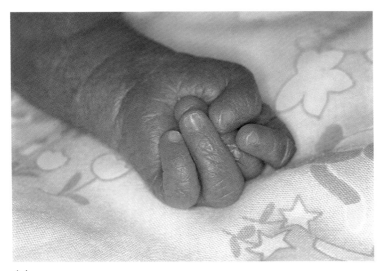

14.

a. What is the diagnosis in this newborn infant?
b. What are the associated findings?
c. What is the prognosis?

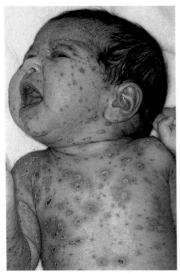

15. The mother of this neonate developed a similar rash a few days before delivery.

a. What is the diagnosis?
b. What is the treatment?
c. What is the prognosis?
d. How could the severity have been reduced?

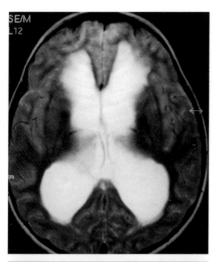

A

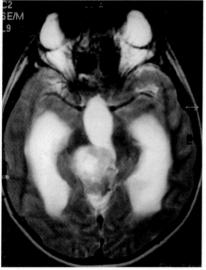

B

16. **These MRI scans are of an 8-year-old boy with headaches and vomiting.**

a. What is the diagnosis?
b. What other clinical signs and symptoms should be looked for?

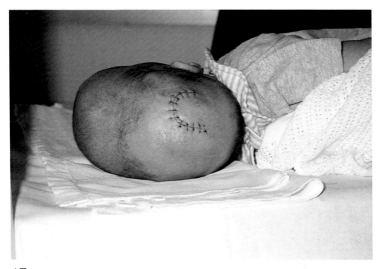

17. **This 4-month-old infant has severe posthaemorrhagic hydrocephalus.**

a. What operation has been performed?
b. What are the complications?

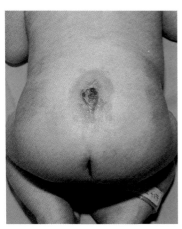

18. **This a newborn infant.**

a. What is the diagnosis?
b. What complications are anticipated?
c. How would one assess the infant clinically?
d. What factors predict severe disability?
e. What antenatal measures can reduce the risk of this condition?

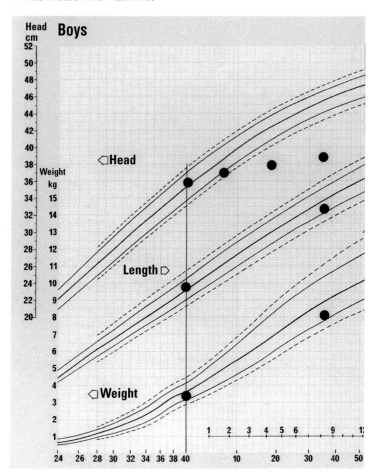

19. This is the growth chart of a 9-month-old boy born at full term with a history of placental abruption and neonatal convulsions.

a. What is demonstrated on the growth chart?
b. What is the likely cause?

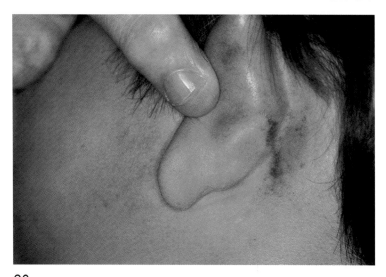

20. **This 3-year-old presented to accident and emergency with bruising.**

a. What is shown?
b. What features of the examination would alert the physician?

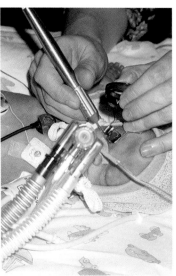

21. **This is a 7-week-old infant born at 25 weeks gestation.**

a. What procedure is being performed?
b. Which infants should be screened at what age?

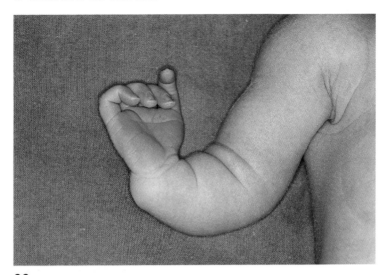

22. This child was born with this abnormality.

a. What is shown?
b. What are the associated conditions?

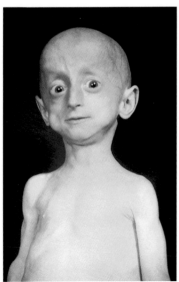

23.

a. What is the diagnosis in this 10-year-old boy?
b. What are the associated features?
c. What is the inheritance?
d. What is the prognosis?

24. The slide shows sputum from a 14-year-old Asian boy with a chronic cough.

a. What is demonstrated in the sputum?
b. What investigations should be performed?
c. What is the management?

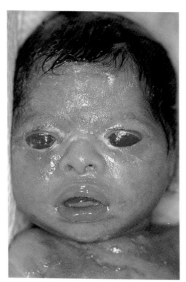

25. This is the face of a newborn infant.

a. What is the differential diagnosis?
b. What is the treatment?

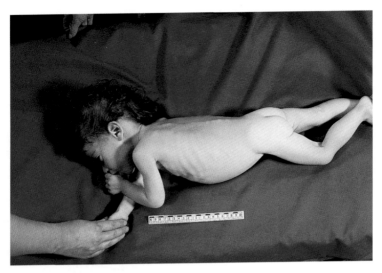

26. This child is aged 6 months.

a. What abnormality is shown?
b. What might be the cause?
c. How would one initially assess the condition?

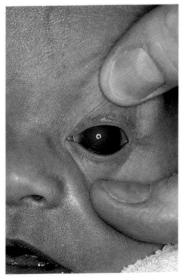

27. This is the eye of a newborn infant.

a. What is the diagnosis?
b. What is the treatment?

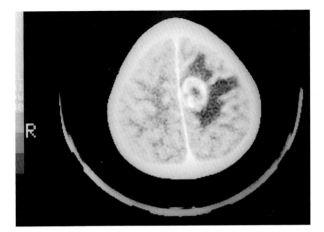

28. Computed tomography (CT) scan of a 6-year-old boy with right-sided focal fits.

a. Describe the abnormality.
b. What is the differential diagnosis?
c. What investigations may be helpful?

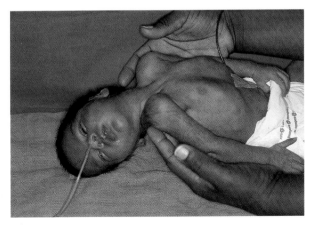

29. This is a term infant aged 2 days.

a. What is shown and what is the differential diagnosis?
b. How would one investigate?

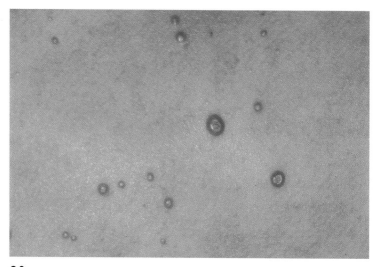

30. This is a photograph from a well 2-year-old.

a. What is the diagnosis?
b. What is the treatment?

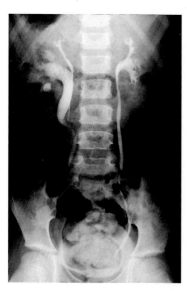

31. This X-ray is of a 5-year-old girl with recurrent urinary tract infections.

a. What is the radiological investigation and what is demonstrated?
b. What other radiological investigations may be helpful?
c. What is the management?

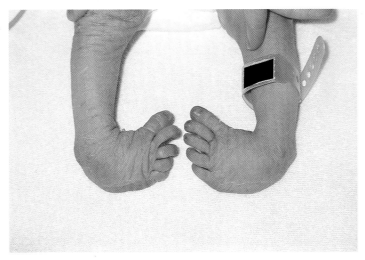

32. These are the feet of a newborn infant.

a. What is the diagnosis?
b. What is the aetiology?
c. What is the treatment?

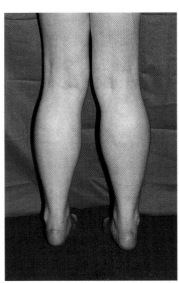

33. This 4-year-old boy has difficulty climbing stairs.

a. What is shown?
b. What is the diagnosis?
c. What are the other features of this condition?
d. How can the diagnosis be confirmed?
e. How is this condition inherited?

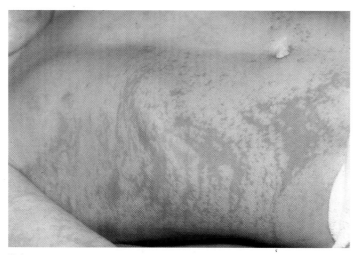

34. This rash started as bullae at birth.

a. What is the diagnosis?
b. What are the associated features?
c. What is the inheritance?

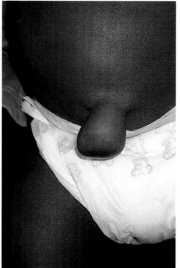

35. This is the umbilicus of a 6-month-old infant.

a. What is the diagnosis?
b. What is the treatment?

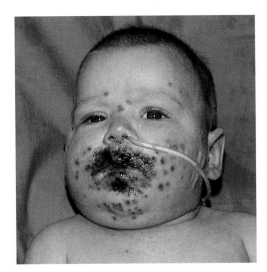

36. This infant presented with refusal to drink.

a. What is the diagnosis?
b. What is the treatment?
c. What is the prognosis?

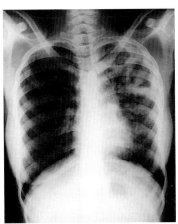

37. This 14-year-old girl has had a persistent cough over 6 months.

a. What is the diagnosis?
b. How can this diagnosis be confirmed?
c. What is the management?

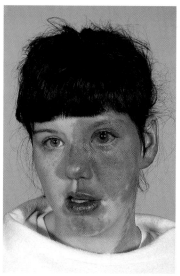

38. This 13-year-old has recurrent fits.

a. What is the diagnosis?
b. Are there ophthalmic complications?
c. What are the associated features?
d. What radiological investigations should be performed?
e. What is the inheritance?

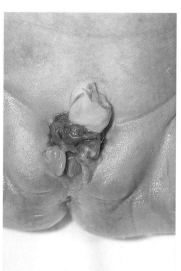

39. This is the anterior abdominal wall of a newborn infant.

a. What is the diagnosis?
b. What is the treatment?

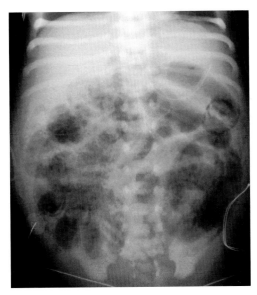

40. This 3-day-old infant with recurrent apnoea had a birth weight of 1760 g at 35 weeks gestation.

a. What does the plain abdominal radiograph show?
b. What is the diagnosis?
c. What other radiological signs may be seen in this condition?

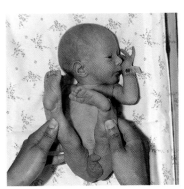

41. This is a newborn infant.

a. What is the diagnosis?
b. What are the complications?
c. What investigation should be performed?

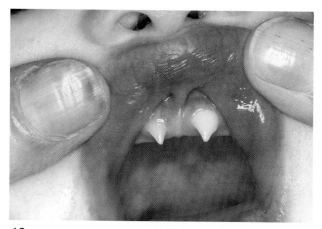

42. **This is the mouth of a 3-year-old male.**

a. What is the diagnosis?
b. What are the associated findings?
c. What is the inheritance?

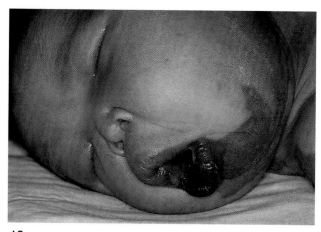

43. **This newborn infant has stridor.**

a. What is the diagnosis?
b. What are the complications?

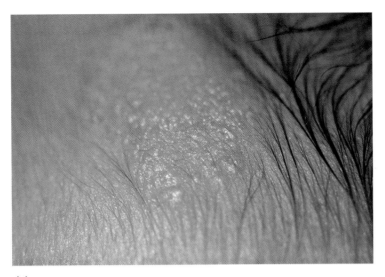

44. This lesion was found on the skin at birth.

a. What is the diagnosis?
b. What are the associated conditions?

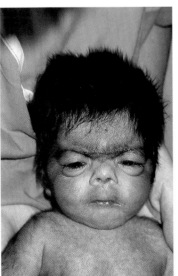

45. This infant had severe feeding difficulties.

a. What is the diagnosis?
b. What are the associated features?
c. What is the inheritance?

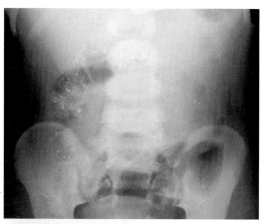

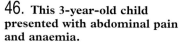

A

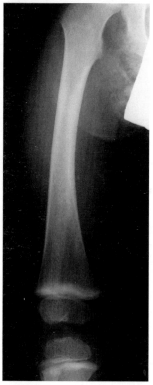

46. This 3-year-old child presented with abdominal pain and anaemia.

a. What abnormalities can be seen on the abdominal X-ray and in the long bones?
b. What is the diagnosis?
c. How would you confirm the diagnosis?

B

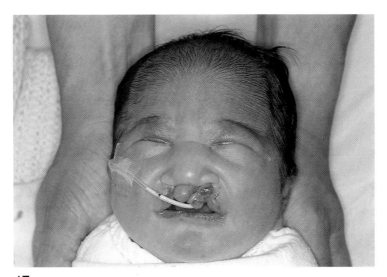

47. This abnormality was present from birth.

a. What is the diagnosis?
b. What are the associated abnormalities?
c. What is the prognosis?

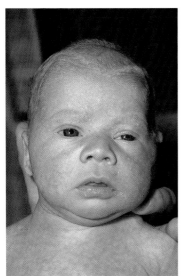

48. This 6-month-old infant presented with lethargy and constipation.

a. What is the diagnosis?
b. What are the associated abnormalities?
c. What investigations should be performed?
d. What is the treatment?
e. What is the prognosis?

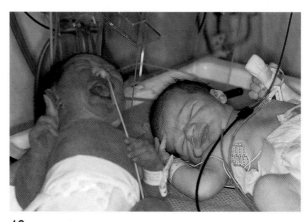

49. This is a pair of newborn twins.

a. What is the diagnosis?
b. What is the zygosity of this pair?
c. What are the complications?

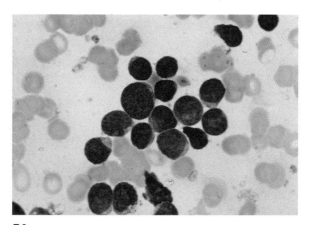

50. The slide shows bone marrow from a 5-year-old child with pallor and bruising.

a. What are the diagnostic features of this bone marrow?
b. What are the useful prognostic indicators in this condition?
c. What are the complications?
d. What is the management and prognosis?

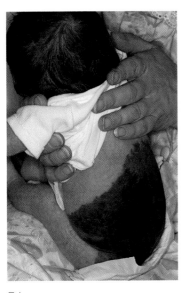
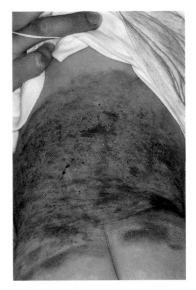

51. **(A) shows a newborn infant and (B) shows the same infant at 6 months of age after treatment.**

a. What is the diagnosis (A)?
b. What are the complications of this condition?
c. What procedure has been performed (B)?

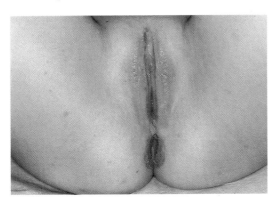

52. **This is the perineum of a 6-year-old girl.**

a. What is the diagnosis?
b. What is the treatment?

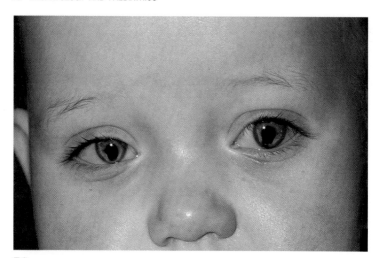

53. This photograph is of a 1-year-old girl.

a. What is the diagnosis?
b. What are the associated findings?

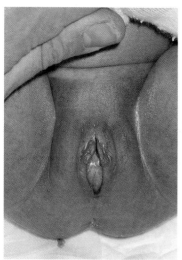

54. This is the perineum of a newborn infant.

a. What is the differential diagnosis?
b. What are the complications?

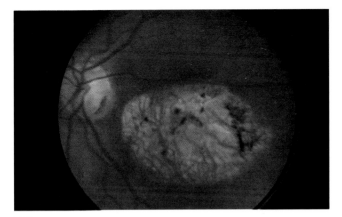

55. This is the retina of a 6-month-old infant.

a. What is the diagnosis?
b. What is the aetiology?
c. What are the complications of this lesion?

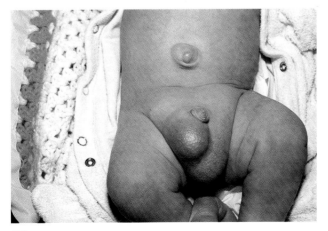

56. This 6-week-old infant presented with vomiting.

a. What is the diagnosis?
b. What is the treatment?

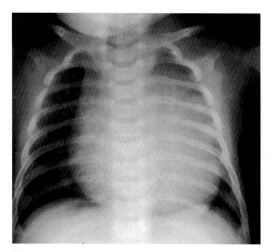

57. This chest X-ray is of a 1-month-old infant with tachypnoea and failure to thrive.

a. What is demonstrated on the chest X-ray?
b. What is the differential diagnosis?
c. What other investigations are likely to be helpful?

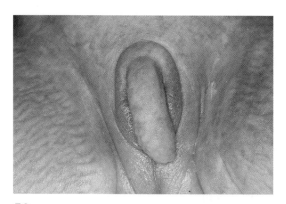

58. The photograph shows the genital appearance of a young infant.

a. What is the diagnosis?
b. What is the treatment?
c. What are the complications?

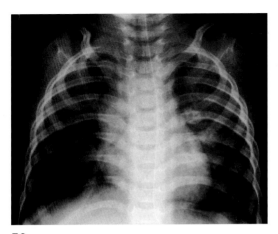

59. This infant, who was born at 24 weeks gestation with a birth weight of 560 g, presented with irritability and tachypnoea at 4 months.

a. What abnormality can be seen on chest X-ray?
b. What is the differential diagnosis?
c. What investigations should be performed?

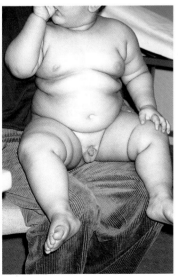

60. This 11-month-old weighs 14 kg.

a. What are the differential diagnoses?
b. What other features help to determine the cause?

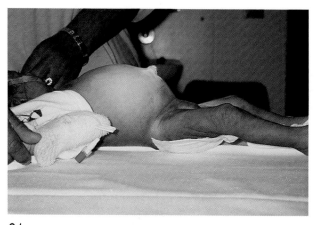

61. This 3-week-old infant presented with delayed passage of stool, failure to thrive and abdominal distension.

a. What is the differential diagnosis?
b. How can this be confirmed?
c. What is the treatment?

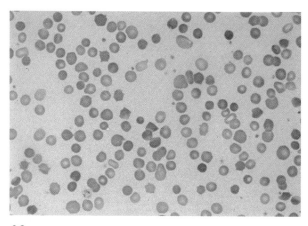

62. This 6-month-old infant had a history of prolonged neonatal jaundice.

a. What is the diagnosis?
b. What are the complications of this condition?
c. What is the management?

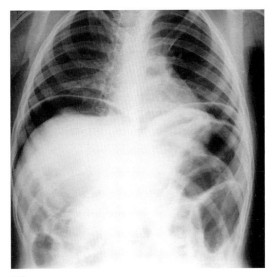

63. **This 8-year-old girl presented with severe abdominal pain.**

a. What is demonstrated?
b. What clinical signs would be present?

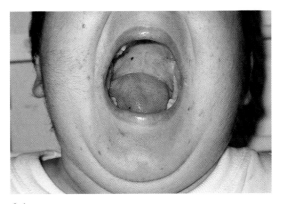

64. **This 10-year-old has been treated for chronic anaemia.**

a. What abnormalities are shown?
b. What is the most likely diagnosis?
c. What treatment options are available?

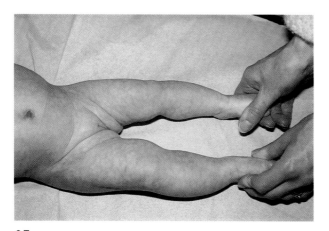

65. This is a 3-month-old girl.

a. What is shown?
b. What is the differential diagnosis?
c. What investigation should be performed?

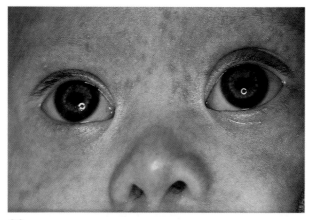

66. This 3-year-old child has developmental delay.

a. What is the diagnosis?
b. What are the associated features?
c. What are the cardiac complications of this condition?

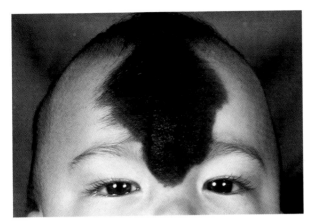

67. This has been present since birth.

a. What is the diagnosis?
b. What are the complications?
c. What is the treatment?

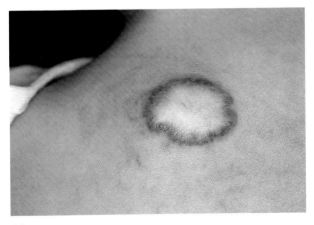

68. This skin lesion developed a few weeks after birth.

a. What is the diagnosis?
b. What is the natural course?
c. What are the complications?

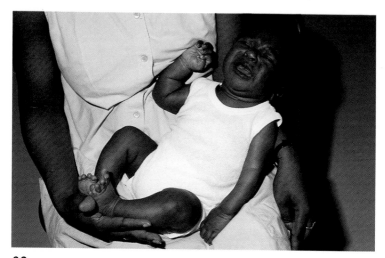

69. This infant suffered shoulder dystocia at his delivery.

a. What is the diagnosis?
b. Where is the lesion?
c. What is the treatment?

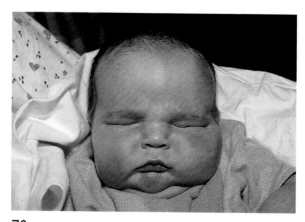

70. This 5 kg baby was admitted to the special care baby unit at age 3 hours with a blood glucose of 0.8 mmol/l.

a. What is the differential diagnosis?
b. What are the complications of these conditions?

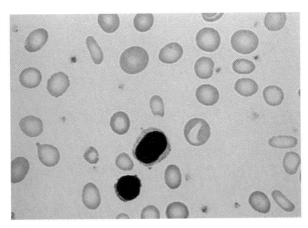

71. This is a peripheral blood film from a 14-month-old child with pallor and poor appetite.

a. What features are shown?
b. What is the differential diagnosis?
c. What clinical information will be helpful in establishing the cause?
d. How would the diagnosis be confirmed?

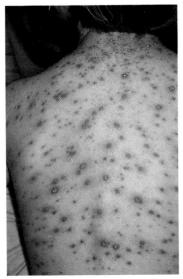

72. This 3-year-old presented with this itchy rash.

a. What is the diagnosis?
b. What is the incubation period?
c. What are the complications?

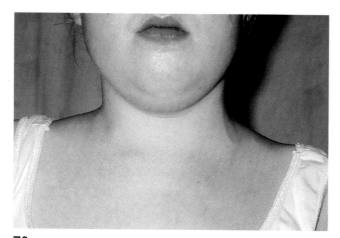

73. **This 10-year-old girl has increasing dyspnoea.**

a. What physical signs can be seen?
b. What is the commonest underlying pathology?
c. What are the dangers from this condition?

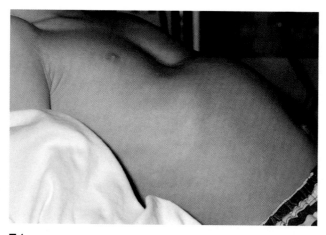

74. **This 3-year-old presented with difficulty in breathing.**

a. What is shown?
b. What is the treatment?

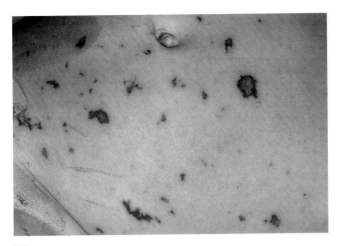

75. This child presented with a fever and a rash.

a. What is the diagnosis?
b. What is the treatment and management?
c. What is the prognosis?
d. What treatment should be offered to the family?

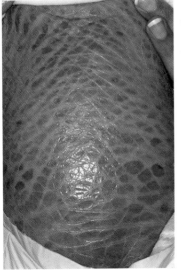

76. This is the skin of a 4-month-old infant.

a. What is the diagnosis?
b. What is the treatment?
c. What is the prognosis?

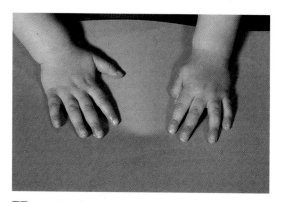

77. **This 18-month-old child presented with delay in walking.**

a. What is the diagnosis?
b. What are the associated physical findings?
c. What investigations should be performed?
d. What is the treatment?

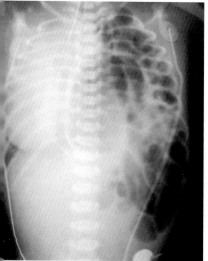

78. **This newborn infant had increasing respiratory distress since birth.**

a. What is the diagnosis and what clinical signs may be present?
b. What is the management of this condition?
c. What is the prognosis?

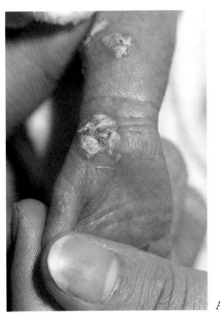

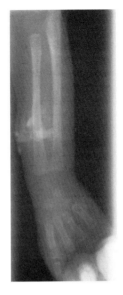

B

A

79. (A) is a photograph from a 7-week-old 25 week gestation infant, and (B) is an X-ray of the arm.

a. What is the differential diagnosis?
b. What is the aetiology?

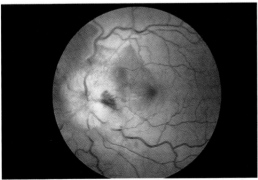

80. This is a retina of a 6-year-old child with a severe headache.

a. What is the diagnosis?
b. What are the causes?

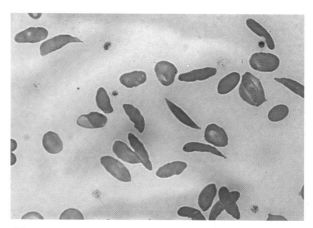

81. This is a peripheral blood film from a 3-year-old Afro-Caribbean child with abdominal pain and mild jaundice.

a. Describe the abnormalities on this blood film.
b. What is the diagnosis?
c. How could the diagnosis be confirmed?
d. What are the common clinical features of this disease?
e. What advice would you give to the family?

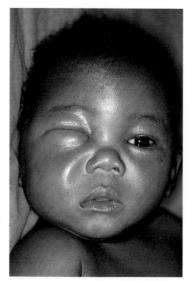

82. This 1-year-old infant presented with fever and malaise.

a. What is the diagnosis?
b. What are the complications?
c. What investigations should be performed?
d. What is the treatment?

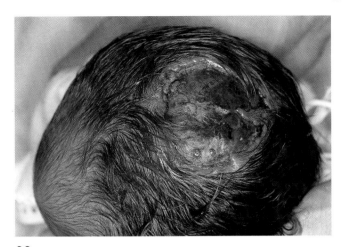

83. This is a newborn infant.

a. What is shown?
b. What are the associated conditions?
c. What investigation should be performed?
d. What is the outcome of this lesion?

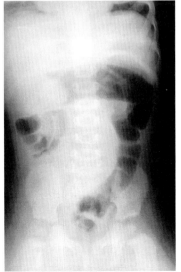

84. This 8-month-old infant presented with sudden onset of vomiting.

a. What investigation has been performed?
b. What is the diagnosis?
c. What other investigations may be helpful in this condition?
d. What is the management?

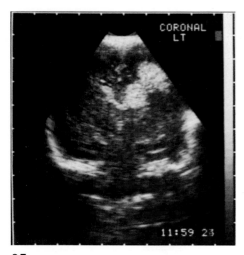

85. **This is a cranial ultrasonography in a 28 week gestation infant at 7 days of age.**

a. What is the diagnosis?
b. What are the clinical features in the first 2 weeks of life?
c. What is the long-term prognosis?

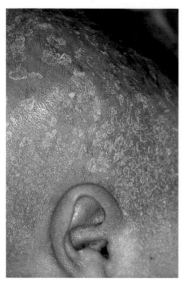

86. **This 3-month-old healthy infant presented with a 1 week history of a rash.**

a. What is the diagnosis?
b. What is the treatment?
c. What is the prognosis?

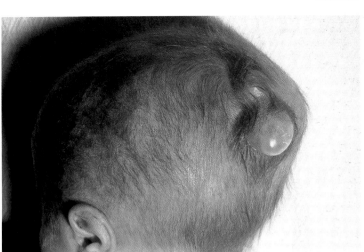

87. This is a newborn infant.

a. What is the differential diagnosis?
b. What is the prognosis?

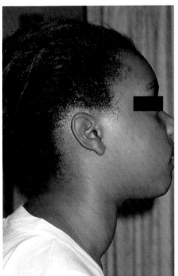

88. This 13-year-old girl had increasing agitation and secondary amenorrhoea.

a. What is shown?
b. What is the differential diagnosis?
c. What is the treatment?

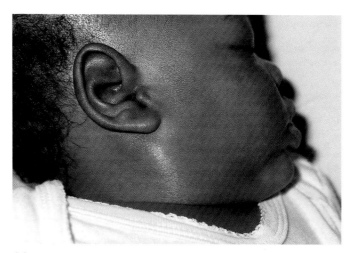

89. This appearance developed after a sore throat.

a. What is the diagnosis?
b. What is the aetiology?
c. What investigations should be performed?
d. What is the treatment?

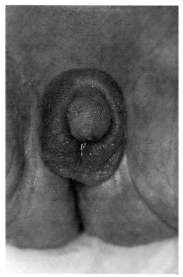

90. This infant presented with vomiting and hyponatraemia at 1 week of age.

a. What is the diagnosis?
b. What investigations are required?
c. What is the treatment?

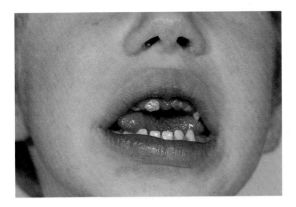

91. This 4-year-old girl had severe constipation.

a. What abnormality is shown?
b. What are the associated features?
c. How should one investigate?
d. Untreated, what is the natural history of this condition?
e. What treatment can be offered?

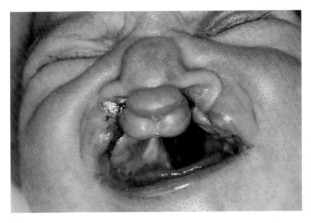

92.

a. What is the diagnosis?
b. What are the associated conditions?
c. What are the complications?
d. What is the treatment?

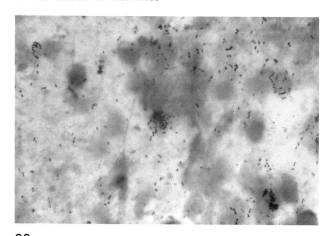

93. Gastric aspirate from a newborn infant who was born at 34 weeks gestation.

a. What is demonstrated?
b. What are the antecedent risk factors which increase the chance of a problem in the infant?
c. Name the common clinical features of this disease.

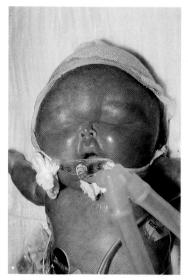

94. This is a preterm infant at 28 weeks gestation.

a. What is the diagnosis?
b. What is the aetiology?
c. What is the treatment?

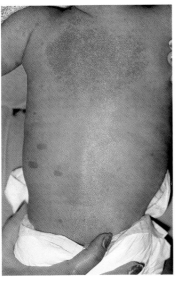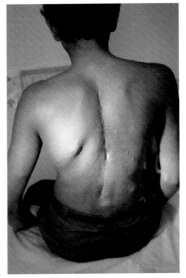

A **B**

95. Both children in these photographs suffer the same condition.

a. What is shown?
b. What is the diagnosis?
c. What are the criteria for diagnosis?
d. How is the condition transmitted?

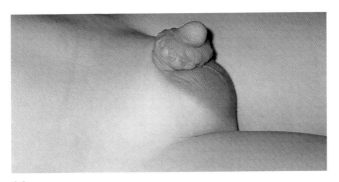

96. This 6-year-old boy presented with a painless swelling of his genitals.

a. What is the diagnosis?
b. What is the treatment?

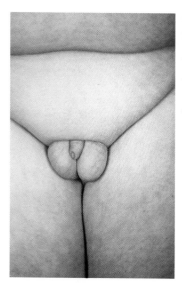

97. This is a 14-year-old obese boy with developmental delay.

a. What is the differential diagnosis?
b. Could these conditions be inherited?
c. What are the other features?

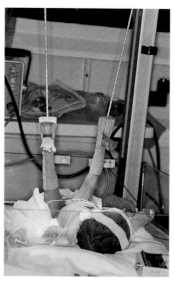

98.

a. What is being shown?
b. Why is it used?

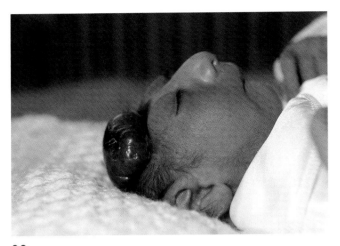

99. This is a newborn infant.

a. What is the diagnosis?
b. What is the prognosis?
c. What advice should be given to the mother regarding future pregnancies?

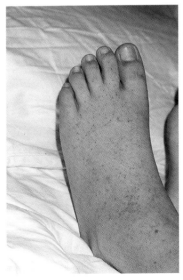

100. This rash appeared in a well child with the following blood count: Hb, 11.0 g/dl; WBC, 7.0 × 10⁹/l; Plat, 22 × 10⁹/l. No abnormal cells were seen on blood film.

a. What is the diagnosis?
b. What further investigations should be performed?
c. What are the indications for bone marrow aspirate?
d. What are the indications for treatment?
e. What is the prognosis?

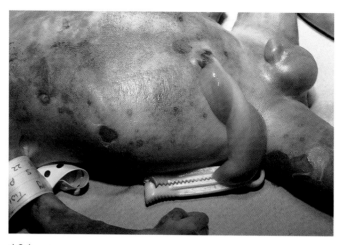

101. This 25 week gestation infant was born in green discoloured liquor and has severe lung disease.

a. What is the differential diagnosis?
b. What urgent investigations should be performed?
c. What is the treatment?

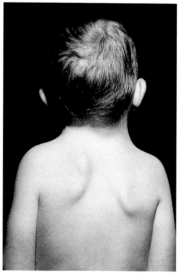

102. This is a 4-year-old boy.

a. What is shown and what is the diagnosis?
b. What is the cause?

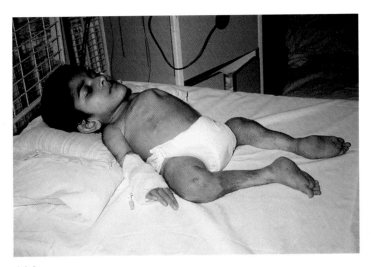

103. This is a 14-year-old boy.

a. What is the diagnosis?
b. What are the associated features?
c. What is the inheritance?

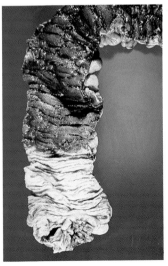

104. This is a pathology specimen, taken at colectomy, demonstrating the ascending colon.

a. Describe the pathological appearance. What is the diagnosis?
b. What is the likely clinical presentation?

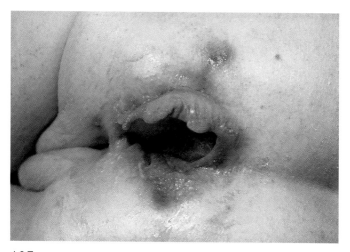

105. This 8-year-old presented with painful defaecation.

a. What is the diagnosis?
b. What are the other presenting symptoms of this condition?
c. What investigations should be performed?
d. What is the treatment?

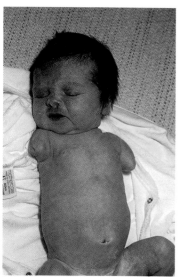

106. This is a newborn infant.

a. What is the diagnosis?
b. What is the treatment?

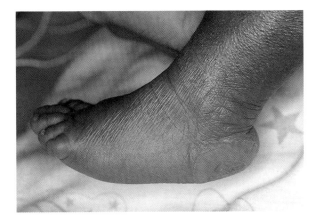

107. **This infant has congenital heart disease.**

a. Describe the abnormality.
b. What is the diagnosis?
c. What are the associated renal abnormalities?

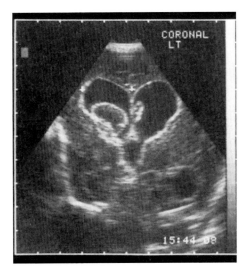

108. **This is a cranial ultrasound in a 3-week-old preterm infant.**

a. Describe the abnormality.
b. What is the diagnosis?
c. What is the management of this condition?

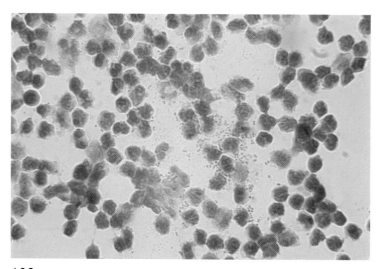

109. The slide shows cerebrospinal fluid (CSF) from an 8-year-old child with a headache, vomiting and photophobia.

a. What is the diagnosis?
b. How can the diagnosis be confirmed?

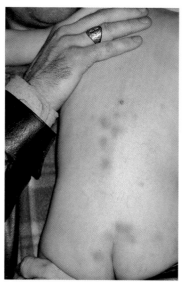

110. This is a 4-year-old boy who presented to the casualty department after these marks were noticed by a nursery school teacher.

a. Wht is the diagnosis?
b. What is characteristic about the distribution of these marks?
c. What features of the history would alert the physician?

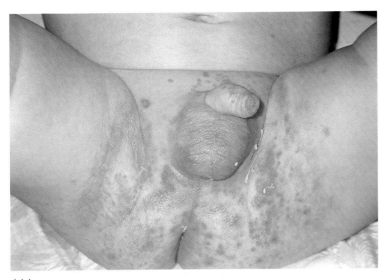

111. This is a well 3-month-old infant.

a. What is the rash?
b. What is the treatment?

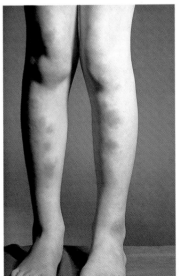

112. This 7-year-old presented with tender lesions on her shins.

a. What is the rash?
b. What is the aetiology?

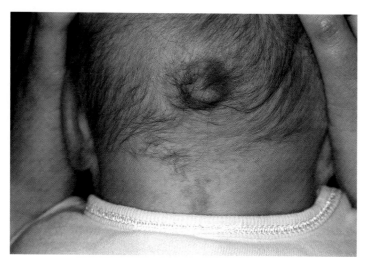

113. **This is a photograph of the occiput from a 1-month-old infant.**

a. What is the diagnosis?
b. What is the management?

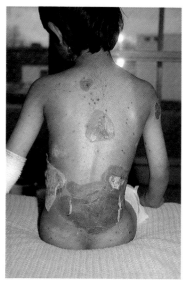

114. **This 6-year-old with chickenpox presented with fever, malaise and widespread skin lesions.**

a. What is the diagnosis?
b. What are the complications?
c. What is the treatment?

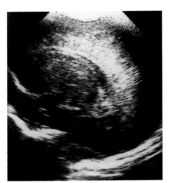

A 3 days

115. (A), (B) and (C) are serial cranial ultrasounds in a preterm infant born at 25 weeks gestation.

a. Describe the findings and the diagnosis.
b. What is the prognosis?

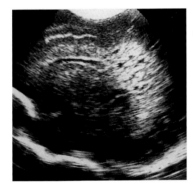

B 18 days

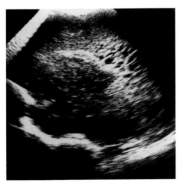

C 26 days

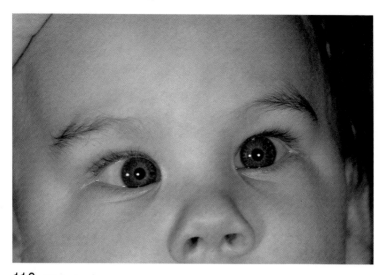

116. This is a 1-year-old infant.

a. What is the diagnosis?
b. What else should one examine?

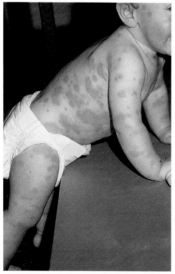

117. This 1-year-old has had an intensely pruritic rash for 3 hours.

a. What is the diagnosis?
b. What are the causes?
c. What are the treatment options?

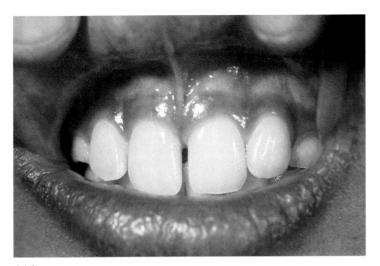

118. This 12-year-old presented with shock and hypoglycaemia.

a. What is shown and what is the diagnosis?
b. What is the treatment?

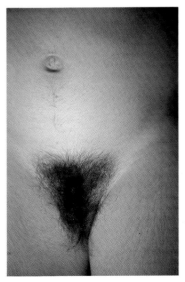

119. This photograph is of a 7-year-old girl.

a. What is the diagnosis?
b. What is the aetiology?
c. What investigations should be performed?

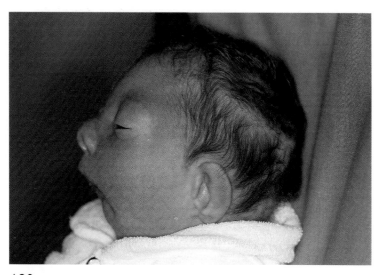

120. This newborn infant had difficulty in breathing.

a. What is the diagnosis?
b. What advice should be given to the parents?

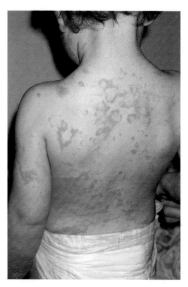

121. This rash has been present for 2 days.

a. What is the diagnosis?
b. What is the cause?
c. What else should one examine?

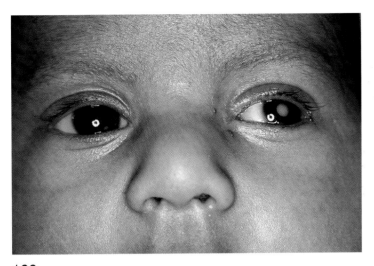

122. This is a 6-month-old infant.

a. What is the diagnosis?
b. What is the aetiology?
c. What is the treatment?

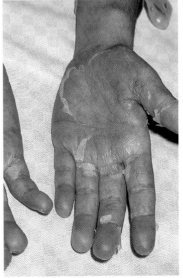

123. This 7-year-old presented after a febrile illness.

a. What is the differential diagnosis?
b. What else should be examined?

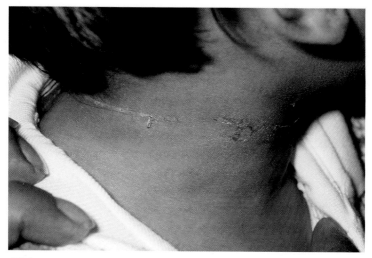

124.

a. What is the diagnosis?
b. During resuscitation, what precaution should be taken?

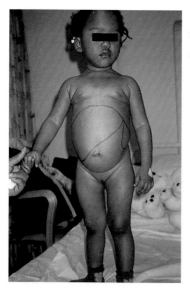

125. This 3-year-old has massive hepatosplenomegaly.

a. What is the differential diagnosis?

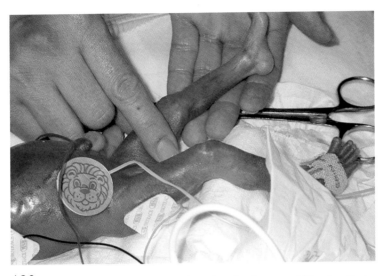

126. This 25 week gestation infant has had an umbilical catheter inserted.

a. What complication is shown?
b. What is the treatment?

127. This child presented with a rash on antibiotic therapy.

a. What is the diagnosis?
b. What is the aetiology?
c. What is the treatment?

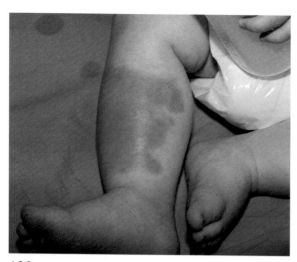

128. This 5-month-old presented with a short history of fever and irritability.

a. What is the diagnosis?
b. What is the likely organism?
c. What are the complications?
d. What is the treatment?

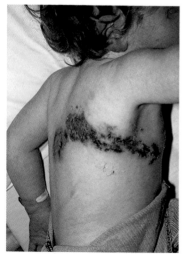

129. This is 4-year-old child.

a. What is the diagnosis?
b. What are the complications?
c. What is the treatment?

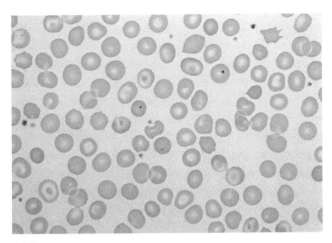

130. This child had an abdominal operation following trauma at the age of 4 years.

a. What features are seen on this peripheral blood film?
b. What is the diagnosis and what are the causes?
c. What are the long-term complications and recommendations?

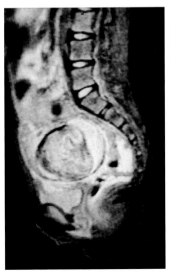

131. This is a magnetic resonance scan of an 11-year-old girl with abdominal pain and increasing abdominal girth.

a. What does the MRI demonstrate?
b. What is the differential diagnosis?

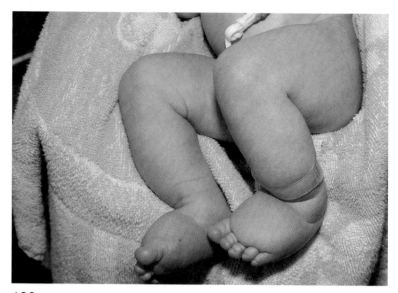

132. This is a newborn female infant.

a. What abnormality is shown?
b. What is the associated condition?
c. What definitive investigation should be performed?
d. What are the associated abnormalities?

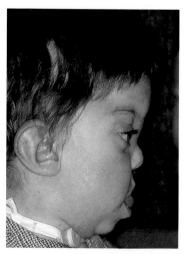

133. This is a 3-year-old boy.

a. What is the diagnosis?
b. What is the treatment?

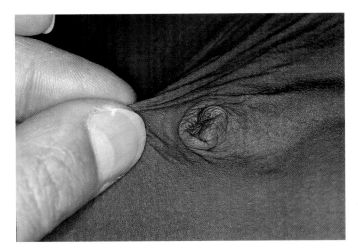

A

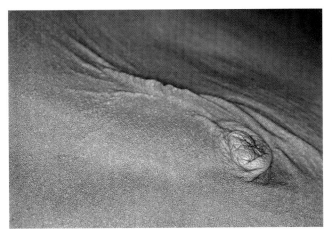

B

134. This previously well 5-year-old presented with profuse diarrhoea and vomiting. (A) shows the skin while it is being lifted, and (B) after it is released.

a. What is the diagnosis and what sign is being demonstrated?
b. How is the clinical severity of this condition described?
c. What is the treatment?

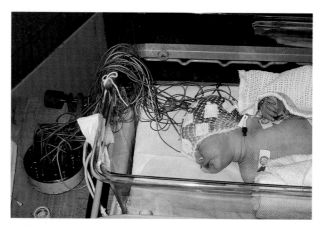

135. **This is a 2-day-old infant who had severe birth asphyxia.**

a. What procedure is being performed?
b. What are the clinical features of hypoxic ischaemic encephalopathy (HIE)?
c. What other investigations would be helpful?

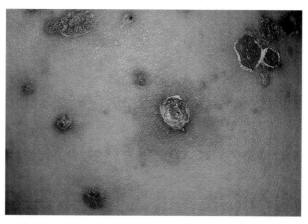

136. **This 4-year-old presented with a rash and fever.**

a. What is the diagnosis?
b. What are the complications?
c. What is the treatment?

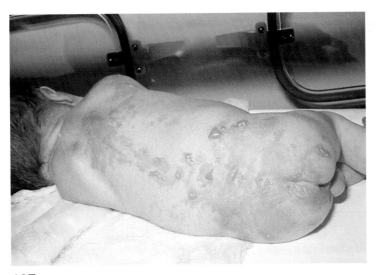

137. This 3-day-old infant developed widespread blistering.

a. What is the diagnosis?
b. What are the variants of this condition?
c. What is the treatment?

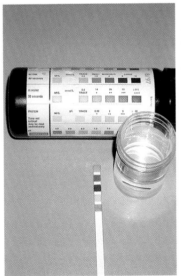

138. This urine sample is from a 5-year-old with weight loss and thirst.

a. What is shown?
b. What is the diagnosis?
c. What is the treatment?

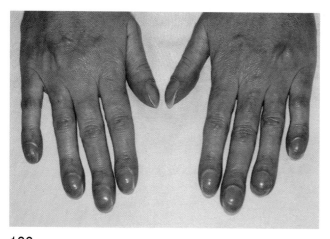

139. These are the hands of a 9-year-old child.

a. What is the diagnosis?
b. What are the causes?

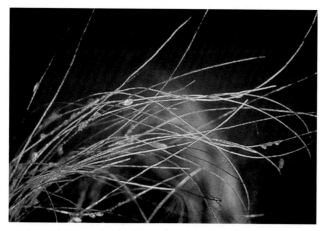

140. This is hair from a 4-year-old.

a. What is the diagnosis?
b. What is the treatment?
c. What other action should be taken?

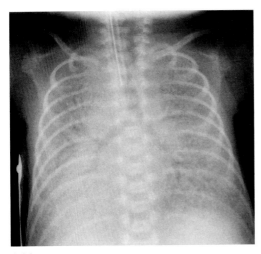

141. This 6-hour-old infant was born at 28 weeks gestation, with a birth weight 1250 g.

a. Describe the radiological features.
b. What is the differential diagnosis?
c. What complications can be demonstrated by radiological investigations?

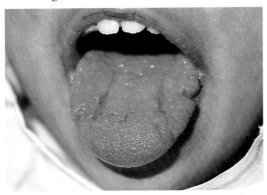

142. This photograph is of a 2-year-old infant.

a. What is shown?
b. What is the differential diagnosis?

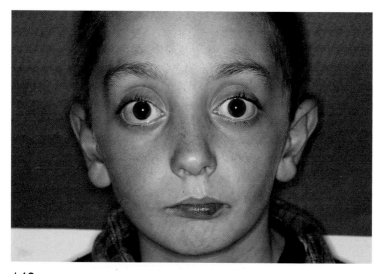

143. **This 7-year-old boy presented with severe headaches.**

a. What physical sign is shown?
b. What is the aetiology?
c. What are the complications?
d. What investigations should be performed?

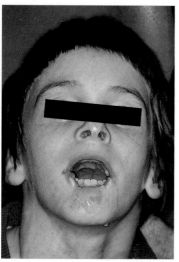

144. **This 9-year-old boy has severe developmental delay.**

a. What is the diagnosis?
b. What are the other features of this condition?
c. What is the underlying defect?
d. How is it inherited?

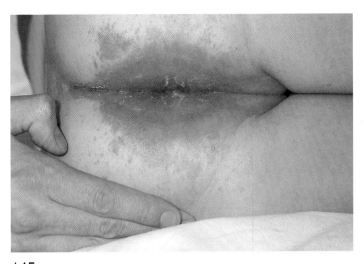

145. This 4-year-old has had perianal discharge for 2 weeks.

a. What is the diagnosis?
b. How can this be confirmed and what is the treatment?
c. What must be excluded?

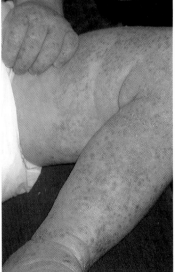

146. This 1-year-old has had this pruritic rash for 3 months.

a. What is the diagnosis?
b. What are the treatment options?
c. What is the role of dietary manipulation?

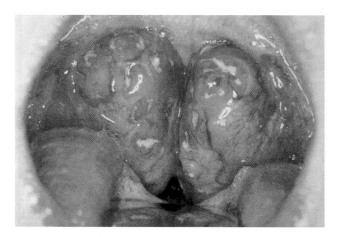

147. This appearance was seen in the oropharynx of a 4-year-old with a fever.

a. What is the diagnosis?
b. What are the complications?
c. What are the indications for surgery?

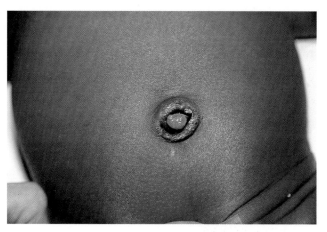

148. This 6-week-old infant has a moist umbilicus.

a. What is the diagnosis?
b. What is the treatment?

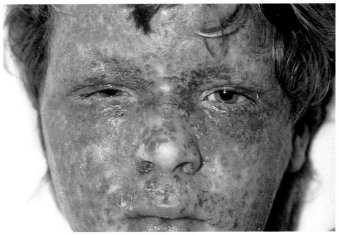

149. This child had moderate eczema which has rapidly deteriorated.

a. What is the diagnosis?
b. What is the treatment?

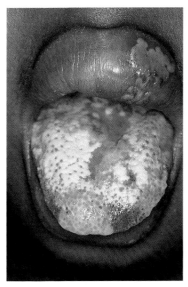

150. This child presented with a sore mouth during chemotherapy.

a. What is the diagnosis?
b. What investigations should be performed?
c. What is the treatment?

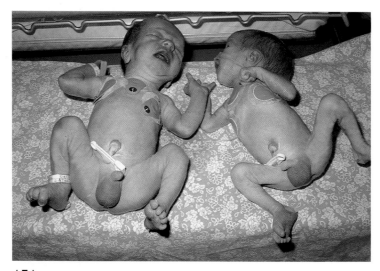

151. Both of these infants are the same gestational age. The infant on the left weighed 3.3 kg at birth.

a. What is the diagnosis for the other infant?
b. What is the aetiology?
c. What problems may occur?

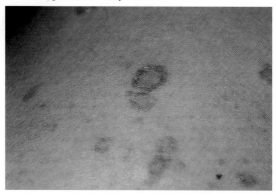

152. This 6-year-old has had this rash for 7 days.

a. What is the diagnosis?
b. What is the treatment?

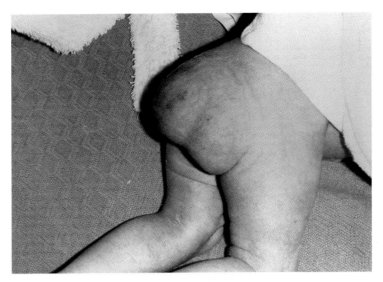

153. This is a newborn infant.

a. What is the diagnosis?
b. What investigations should be performed?
c. What is the prognosis?

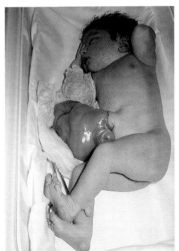

154. This is a newborn infant.

a. What is the diagnosis?
b. What are the associated abnormalities?
c. What is the treatment?

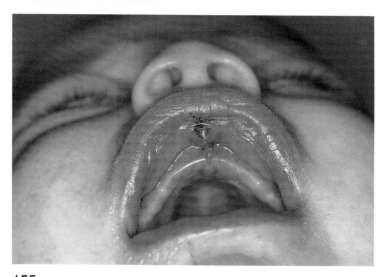

155. This is the mouth of a 6-month-old.

a. What is the lesion shown?
b. What should the clincan consider?

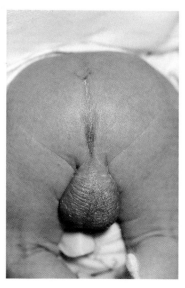

156. This is a newborn boy.

a. What is the diagnosis?
b. What are the associated abnormalities?
c. How is this treated?

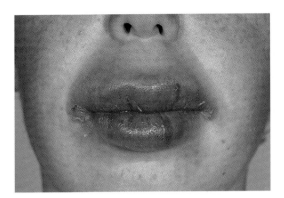

157. This well 12-year-old presented with recurrent abdominal pain.

a. What signs are shown and what is the diagnosis?
b. What is the treatment?

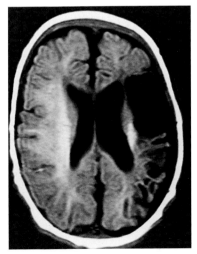

158. This is an MRI scan of a 4-month-old infant who had neonatal convulsions.

a. Describe the abnormal findings.
b. What is the diagnosis?
c. What is the prognosis?

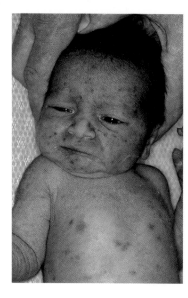

159. **This newborn term infant has a birth weight of 2.2 kg and hepatosplenomegaly.**

a. What is the diagnosis?
b. What are the associated features of this condition?
c. How can the diagnosis be confirmed?

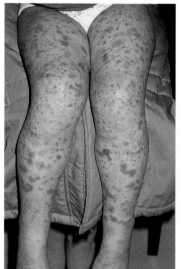

160. **This a well 5-year-old presenting with abdominal pain.**

a. What is the diagnosis?
b. What are the manifestations of this condition?
c. What is the treatment?

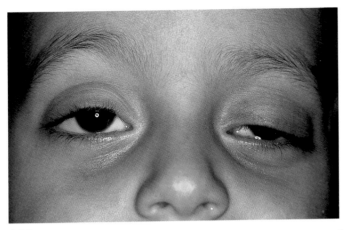

161. This 6-year-old girl presented with a short history of double vision and difficulty in lifting her arm.

a. What is shown?
b. What is the diagnosis?
c. How would this be confirmed?
d. What is the treatment?

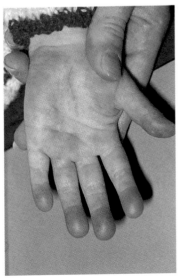

162. This 1-year-old presented with persistent fever, conjunctivitis and cervical lymphadenopathy.

a. What is the diagnosis?
b. What are the criteria for diagnosis?
c. What are the complications?
d. What is the treatment?

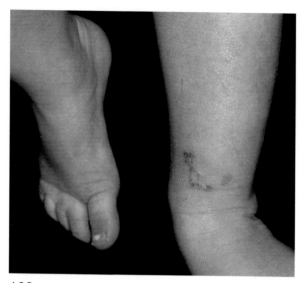

163. This 2-year-old girl had an intensively pruritic lesion since returning from the West Indies, which failed to improve on topical steroids or antibiotics.

a. What is the diagnosis?
b. What is the treatment?

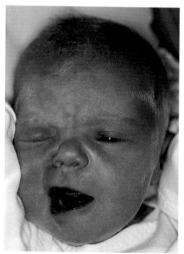

164. This is a newborn infant.

a. What is the diagnosis?
b. What is the aetiology?
c. What are the prognosis and treatment?

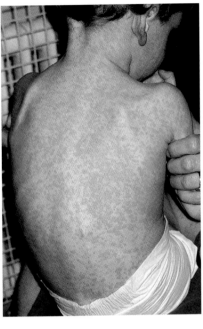

165. This 4-year-old presented with a rash after taking ampicillin for sore throat and lymphadenopathy.

a. What is the diagnosis?
b. What is the causative organism?
c. What are the complications of the underlying condition?

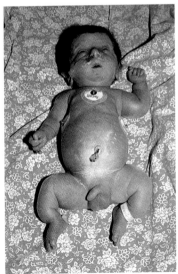

166. This is a newborn infant.

a. What is the diagnosis?
b. What is the prognosis?

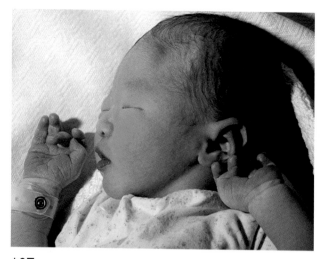

167. This is a newborn infant.

a. What is the diagnosis?
b. What investigation should be performed?

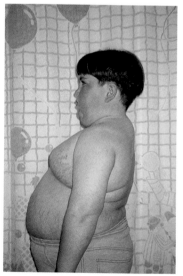

168. This is a 12-year-old boy.

a. What physical signs are shown?
b. What is the diagnosis?
c. What are the causes?
d. What investigations should be performed?

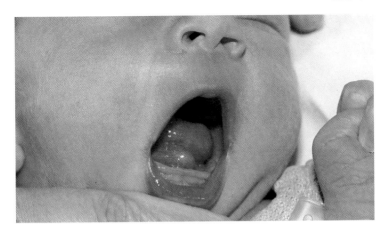

169. This is the mouth of a newborn infant.

a. What is the diagnosis?
b. What is the prognosis?

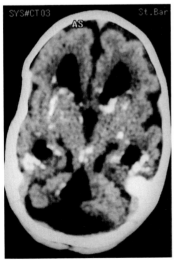

170. This is a CT scan of a newborn infant with microcephaly.

a. What abnormalities are shown?
b. What is the differential diagnosis?
c. What are the other features of these conditions?

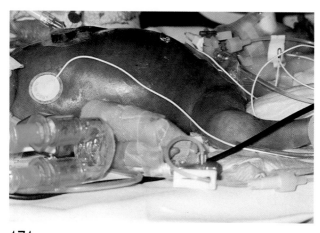

171. This is a 10-day-old neonate born at 26 weeks gestation.

a. What is the diagnosis?
b. What are early signs of this condition?
c. What are the risk factors for this condition?
d. What is the treatment?
e. What is the prognosis?

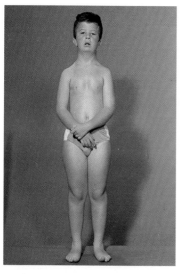

172. This 7-year-old has short stature and a heart murmur.

a. What is the diagnosis?
b. What are the associated abnormalities?
c. How is this inherited?

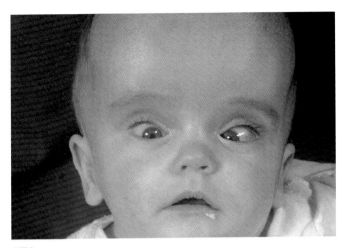

173. This child has had an increasing head circumference since birth.

a. What is the diagnosis, and what features are shown?
b. What is the aetiology?

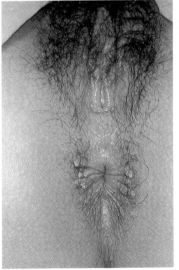

174. This 12-year-old presented with bleeding from the anus.

a. What is the diagnosis?
b. What should the clinician suspect?
c. How should the clinician proceed?

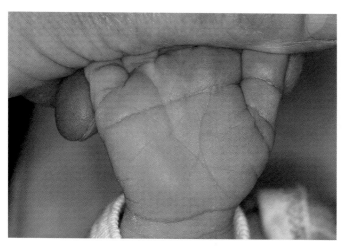

175.

a. What abnormality is shown?
b. What are the associated conditions?
c. What other hand abnormalities occur in these conditions?

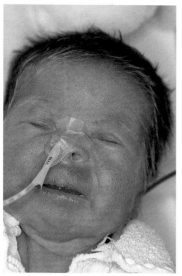

176. **This is a 1-day-old infant.**

a. What is the diagnosis?
b. What is the aetiology?
c. What are the immediate investigations?
d. What is the treatment?

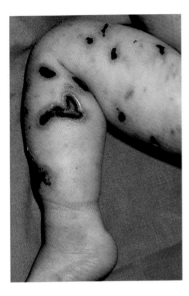

177. This 18-month-old presented in a collapsed state.

a. What is the diagnosis?
b. What is the differential aetiology?
c. What is the treatment?

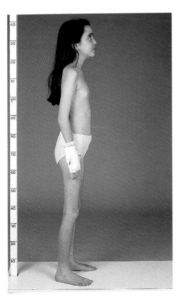

178. This is a 15-year-old girl.

a. What physical signs are demonstrated?
b. What are the causes?
c. What assessment should be performed?

Answers

1.
   a. Hypospadias—urethral meatus opening on the ventral aspect of the glans.
   b. Hypospadius is usually an isolated abnormality. Chordee, undescended tests and other genitourinary anomalies are sometimes associated. Renal and bladder ultrasound should be performed in patients with a severe proximal hypospadius.
   c. Circumcision should be delayed until surgical repair is completed as the prepuce may be required for urethroplasty. Surgery may be needed to correct the chordee.

2.
   a. Psoriasis—plaques with scaling and erythema typically on the trunk, elbows and knees.
   b. Associated with pitting of nails, oncholysis and psoriatic arthropathy, not commonly involving distal interphalangeal joints.
   c. Topical therapy includes topical salicylic acid, dithranol, coal tar or vitamin D analogues (e.g. calcipotriol). A course of ultraviolet light therapy (UVB) may be helpful. Treat streptococcal throat infection if suspected.

3.
   a. Juvenile chronic arthritis (JCA), systemic lupus erythematosus (SLE). Other causes of childhood arthritis include reactive arthritis, Henoch–Schönlein purpura, septic arthritis, rheumatic fever and inflammatory bowel disease.
   b. Other features include:
- JCA—arthropathy, fever, lymphadenopathy, macular rash, anaemia, hepatosplenomegaly and growth failure. Uveitis may be present in pauciarticular JCA
- SLE—arthropathy, butterfly rash, fever, malaise, Raynaud phenomena, neuropsychiatric symptoms and nephropathy.

   c. Activity and exercise should be maintained whenever possible. Physiotherapy, hydrotherapy and splinting provide symptomatic relief and reduce the disability. Non-steroidal anti-inflammatory drugs such as aspirin, indomethacin or ibuprofen relieve symptoms. Corticosteroids and immunomodulatory drugs may be required in a small minority of cases.

4.
   a. Choanal atresia—note the oral airway and orogastric tube.
   b. Usually an isolated lesion but may be part of CHARGE syndrome complex—coloboma, heart disease (varying from Fallot's tetralogy to persistent ductus arteriosus), atresia

choanae, **r**enal anomalies or **r**etarded growth, **g**enital hypoplasia and **e**ar anomalies. Two of these features must be present to make the definitive diagnosis. CHARGE is also associated with learning disability and abnormal facial features such as palatal defects and small mandible. Most cases are isolated, but both autosomal recessive and dominant inheritance have been described.

c. Initially treat with a secured airway as shown. Definitive surgery involves transnasal or transpalatal surgical or laser correction of atresia.

5.
a. Milia—tiny cysts arising from pilosebaceous follicles or sweat ducts.
b. None; they spontaneously disappear over the first months.

6.
a. Trisomy 21—Down syndrome.
b. *Screening* for Down syndrome can be performed by measuring elevated maternal serum βhCG and low α feto protein (double testing), plus oestrodial (triple testing). *Definitive* testing can be performed by karyotyping of cells from amniocentesis or chorionic villous biopsy.
c. There is an increased incidence of atresiae, e.g. tracheo-oesophageal fistula, duodenal atresia, jejunal atresia, duodenal web and Hirschprung's disease.

7.
a. Natal teeth—mandibular central incisors found at birth. They are usually supernumerary, but should be differentiated from prematurely erupted primary teeth before extraction. Note the white coating of the tongue, which is either milk or candida infection; this can be differentiated clinically by testing whether it can be easily removed by gentle rubbing (milk rubs off easily).
b. Pain for the nursing mother, risk of detachment and aspiration of the tooth or tongue laceration. They may require careful extraction. This will not deplete the permanent dentition.

8.
a. McCune–Albright syndrome.
b. Precocious puberty, café au lait pigmentation, classically with an irregular border, and polyostotic fibrous dysplasia (fibrous tissue replacing bone in long bones and pelvis, leading to deformity and pathological fractures). This syndrome is also associated with gigantism, hyperthyroidism, Cushing syndrome and ovarian cysts.
c. Café au lait spots are features of neurofibromatosis type 1, tuberose sclerosis, Bloom syndrome and ataxia telangiectasia.

9.
a. This slide shows a hyperextensible metacarpophalangeal joint of the thumb (passive apposition of the thumb to the flexor

aspect of the forearm). This may occur in isolation but is a feature of Ehlers–Danlos syndrome, a genetically heterogenous connective tissue disorder of variable severity.

b. Affected children appear normal at birth. The most striking features are hyperextensibility, fragility and easy bruising of the skin, resulting in recurrent ecchymoses, bleeding and poor healing. Severe joint hypermobility may lead to skeletal deformity. The condition should be distinguished from cutis laxa in which there is laxity of the skin but no musculoskeletal manifestations.

c. There is no specific treatment and life expectancy is usually normal. Orthopaedic management with braces and physiotherapy may improve musculoskeletal function, and surgery may be indicated to correct vascular abnormalities.

10.
a. Scald to the face.
b. Assess the airway, breathing and circulation. Then assess the burn—surface area, depth and areas involved. Determine the cause and circumstances.
c. Analgesia and fluid replacement are the mainstay of therapy. Scalds to the face may be best managed without dressings but with careful attention to treat infection.

11.
a. Mongolian Blue spot—lumbosacral pigmented macular lesions occurring in a high proportion of black, oriental and Indian infants, and infants of mixed ethnic origin.
b. They become less obvious in the first years of life, and therefore no treatment is required.

12.
a. This is a micturating cystourethrogram demonstrating bilateral grade IV vesicoureteric reflux. There is reflux up grossly distended and tortuous ureters into the pelvic calyceal system, with marked dilatation on the left.
b. A renal ultrasound would usually have been performed before this investigation and would have compared the size of both kidneys and excluded hydronephrosis. A 2,3-dimercaptosuccinic acid (DMSA) scan should be performed to compare renal function on both sides and identify renal scars.
c. Recurrent urinary tract infections in the presence of severe vesicoureteric reflux may lead to renal scarring, especially under the age of 5 years. Prophylactic antibiotics usually prevent recurrent urinary tract infections, and vesicoureteric reflux may improve with age. Renal scarring rarely occurs after the age of 5 years. If there is breakthrough infection, or if prophylactic antibiotics are not acceptable, then surgical reimplantation of the ureters may be required. A repeat

DMSA scan should be performed before discontinuing antibiotic prophylaxis.

13.
a. Short-limbed dwarfism. The most likely diagnosis is thanatophoric dysplasia. Achondroplasia has a similar physical and radiological appearance to the limbs, but the small pear-shaped thorax and hypoplastic lungs make thanatophoric dysplasia lethal at birth.

b. Thanatophoric dysplasia is an autosomal recessive condition. Achondroplasia is inherited as an autosomal dominant trait, but about 80% of cases are new mutations.

14.
a. Trisomy 18—Edward syndrome. This photograph shows clinodactyly, with the second finger overlapping the third.

b. Prominent occiput, small palpebral fissure, narrow nose, narrow bifrontal diameter, micrognathia, low set malformed ears, cleft lip/palate, facial palsy, hirsuitism, short sternum, pulmonary hypoplasia, limited hip abduction, hypoplastic nails, rocker-bottom feet, developmental delay and growth retardation. 95% of cases have congenital heart disease, e.g. ventricular septal defects, persistent ductus arteriosus and atrial septal defects.

c. The majority die within the first few weeks. Few survive beyond 1 year of age.

15.
a. Neonatal chickenpox (transplacentally acquired). Risks to the fetus and neonate from maternal chickenpox are related to the time of infection in the mother. In the first 20 weeks of pregnancy, varicella may result in congenital varicella syndrome, with limb hypoplasia, microcephaly, cataracts, growth retardation and skin scarring. Infection around delivery can result in neonatal chickenpox.

b. The infant should be admitted to hospital. Treatment includes the use of high-dose intravenous acyclovir and aggressive management of pneumonitis and secondary sepsis.

c. Since the chickenpox is transplacentally acquired, there will be viraemia secondary to mother's infection before specific IgG has crossed the placenta. The condition is severe and carries a high mortality, especially if the infant develops pneumonitis.

d. Maternal chickenpox where the rash appears more than 5 days before delivery enables anti-zoster IgG to cross the placenta and protect the neonate. If the maternal rash appears between 7 days prior to delivery and 28 days post-delivery, the baby requires intramuscular zoster immunoglobulin (VZIG) within 48 hours. The baby may still develop chickenpox but the disease should be less severe.

Fatal cases have been reported despite VZIG prophylaxis, when the onset of maternal chickenpox is in the period 4 days before to 2 days after delivery. Early treatment with intravenous acyclovir is recommended for infants in this exposure category who develop varicella despite VZIG prophylaxis.

16.
a. Large brain tumour causing marked ventricular dilatation. Note that the cerebrospinal fluid is represented by white opacification on an MRI scan, but is a dark translucency on a CT scan.
b. Early morning headaches, irritability and vomiting are usually the earliest symptoms, but the diagnosis is often difficult to make in the early stages. Head tilt and ataxia are often seen in young children with posterior fossa tumours. Fundoscopy may reveal signs of papilloedema, with blurring of the optic disc margins and loss of physiological cupping. Cranial nerve palsies and exophthalmos are also seen in tumours diagnosed at a later stage.

17.
a. Rickham reservoir or ventriculoperitoneal shunt to drain cerebrospinal fluid.
b. Complications are:
  - bacterial colonisation of the reservoir or shunt; the most likely organism is coagulase-negative staphylococcus
  - blocking requiring revision of shunt
  - dislocation of shunt tubing
  - over-drainage of cerebrospinal fluid leading to slit-shaped ventricles
  - subdural effusion.

18.
a. Lumbar meningomyelocele.
b. At the lumbar level, complications include lower motor neurone signs in the legs, bladder and rectal sphincter dysfunction, kyphosis, dislocated hips and hydrocephalus.
c. Measure the head circumference and look for clinical evidence of hydrocephalus, e.g. widening of sutures or setting sun sign. Examine the size and level of the defect and determine sensory and motor levels, anal and urinary sphincter function. Examine the hips to assess for dislocation and note any other limb abnormality, e.g. talipes equinovarus.
d. Severe disability is more likely in the presence of gross hydrocephalus at birth, severe paralysis of the lower limbs, kyphosis or scoliosis, incontinence of urine and faeces, abnormality of lower limbs such as talipes and dislocated

hips, and other major congenital defects. Lumbar lesions are associated with more severe disability than thoracic lesions, as the latter are frequently meningoceles.

e. Prenatal (0.4 mg) folic acid daily prior to conception and in the first 12 weeks of pregnancy reduces the incidence of neural tube defects by two-thirds. Screening by measuring maternal serum α feto protein and detailed ultrasound at 13–18 weeks gestation can diagnose the condition antenatally, and termination of pregnancy is then possible.

19.
a. There was good intrauterine growth, but the head circumference has fallen from the 50th centile to far below the 3rd centile.
b. Severe hypoxic ischaemic insult related to the placental abruption.

20.
a. Finger pinch injury to the pinna. This injury is pathognomonic of non-accidental injury.
b. Unexplained bruising, scalds, multiple injuries or bruises of different ages, cigarette burns, bite marks, injuries to the perineum, bruises to pinna, grip marks to face or limbs, failure to thrive, signs of neglect, retinal haemorrhages, deteriorating level of consciousness suggestive of intracranial injury, or bony injury.

21.
a. This photograph shows a ventilated neonate receiving cryotherapy for retinopathy of prematurity (ROP). This condition is the commonest cause of visual impairment acquired in the neonatal period and results from abnormal neovascularisation of the retina. Cryotherapy and laser therapy have been shown to be effective in infants requiring treatment and reduce the incidence of visual impairment.
b. All infants ≤31 weeks gestational age or birth weight <1500 g should be screened for ROP every 2 weeks from 6 weeks postnatal age. This should continue until at least 36 weeks corrected gestational age.

22.
a. Absent radius and thumb.
b. This is associated with cardiac abnormalities and blood dyscrasias, e.g. Radial aplasia—thrombocytopenia syndrome (TAR), Holt–Oram syndrome, Fanconi pancytopenia syndrome, VACTERL association. The VACTERL association is diagnosed when three of seven possible abnormalities are present: **v**ertebral abnormalities, **a**nal atresia, **c**ongenital heart disease, **t**racheal defects, **r**enal abnormalities, absent **r**adius and **l**ung hypoplasia.

23.
a. Progeria (premature ageing).
b. Alopecia, thin skin, hypoplasia of nails and loss of subcutaneous fat, periarticular fibrosis leading to stiff and flexed joints, short stature, facial hypoplasia with micrognathia, and slim tubular bones.
c. This is a sporadic condition. It is extremely rare.
d. Patients die in early adult life from coronary heart disease secondary to generalised atherosclerosis and elevated plasma cholesterol.

24.
a. Ziehl–Neelsen stain demonstrating the typical acid fast bacilli of *Mycobacterium tuberculosis*. The mycobacteria appear red and are typically slender and slightly curved.
b. At this age, the chest X-ray may reveal the typical appearance seen in adults with post-primary tuberculosis (TB), with widespread caseation and cavity formation. In younger children with primary TB, minor enlargement of regional lymph nodes may be the only radiological sign. A positive intradermal tuberculin test (e.g. Mantoux or Heaf test) is likely to be associated with active infection, but the response may be reduced in miliary TB, malnutrition, TB meningitis and in young infants less than 6 weeks of age. Culture of *Mycobacterium tuberculosis* from sputum confirms the diagnosis, but sputum is often difficult to obtain in young children. Gastric washings are also difficult to obtain and are only occasionally helpful.
c. Combination anti-TB chemotherapy is given for at least 6 months. Close contacts of the index case should be screened by chest X-ray and Mantoux or Heaf test. Siblings aged less than 5 years of a sputum-positive index patient are usually given prophylactic anti-TB therapy for 6 months. Long-term follow-up of all childhood cases of TB and close siblings is mandatory.

25.
a. Bilateral ectropion, flattening of the ears and nose, and fish-mouth. These are features of a 'collodion baby', the neonatal manifestation of ichthyosis which comprises a group of inherited keratinizing disorders. In severe cases, the infant may be encased in a shiny brownish membrane which may cause respiratory embarrassment—the 'harlequin fetus'. These infants die within the neonatal period.
b. Treatment comprises intensive skin care with frequent emollient application, baths and keratolytics, and the infant needs to be maintained in a high humidity environment. Fluid and electrolyte balance should be carefully maintained. Special attention needs to be paid to the ectropion, with

careful nursing to avoid secondary infection. Complications of ectropion include corneal ulceration.

26.
a. Failure to thrive (FTT):
- wasted buttocks
- loss of subcutaneous tissues
- abdominal distension
- reduced muscle bulk.

b. The most common cause is inadequate nutritional intake. Almost every chronic and serious condition in childhood may cause FTT. Other causes include:
- feeding problems—technique, inability to suck or swallow
- malabsorption
- cystic fibrosis
- immunodeficiency
- neurological disease
- inflammatory disease
- chromosomal disorders
- other chronic disorders, e.g. renal failure, heart disease
- psychosocial—formula preparation, emotional deprivation, neglect.

c. Detailed history, including neonatal course, feeding and dietary assessment, associated symptoms, e.g. diarrhoea, recurrent infections. Plot height, weight, head circumference and previous measurements on centile charts.

27.
a. Congenital glaucoma. Proptosis with corneal opacification, a watering eye and photophobia. Neonatal retinoblastoma may have a similar appearance.

b. Urgent ophthalmological intervention is required to prevent enlargement of the globe and visual loss.

28.
a. There is a well demarcated circular lesion with an area of central lucency surrounded by an extensive radiolucent area of oedema in the left cerebral hemisphere.

b. Cerebral abscess, bacterial or tuberculous (TB), or a cerebral tumour.

c. Chest X-ray, Mantoux or Heaf test, culture of sputum, urine and gastric washings may confirm the diagnosis of TB. In a febrile and toxic child, blood cultures, peripheral blood leucocytosis and elevated ESR or CRP should be sought. Aspiration or excision biopsy of the lesion may be necessary if other non-invasive investigations do not reveal the diagnosis. In this case, none of the above investigations confirmed a diagnosis, but there was a good response to long-term intravenous broad-spectrum antibiotics including metronidazole.

29.
a. Floppy infant with a nasogastric tube. The differential diagnosis includes hypoxic ischaemic encephalopathy, congenital myotonic dystrophy, congenital myopathies, neonatal myasthenia, intracranial haemorrhage, chromosomal disorders, metabolic disorders and spinal muscular atrophy.
b. Creatine phosphokinase, ultrasound of the muscles, muscle biopsy, nerve conduction velocity, electromyography and intracranial imaging.

30.
a. Molluscum contagiosum—smooth translucent papules with a central punctum caused by pox virus.
b. No treatment is indicated in the majority of cases, as the lesions are asymptomatic. If the lesions are widespread, cryotherapy or needling may reduce the duration. They spontaneously regress within months.

31.
a. This is an intravenous urogram demonstrating a normal left ureter and a duplex right ureter, with dilatation and tortuosity of the lower moiety. There is blunting of the calyces on the right.
b. An indirect radioisotope cystogram (MAG3 isotope) would assess the differential renal function and can detect vesicoureteric reflux. In a younger patient, a 2,3-dimercaptosuccinic acid (DMSA) scan and a direct voiding cystourethrogram (micturating cystourethrogram) should be performed.
c. Vesicoureteric reflux in the presence of duplex ureter rarely settles spontaneously. Long-term prophylactic antibiotics may protect from further infection. Surgery may be necessary if there are recurrent urinary tract infections, or if long-term prophylaxis is not acceptable to the patient.

32.
a. Bilateral congenital talipes equinovarus—the entire foot is inverted and supinated, and the forefoot is adducted.
b. Intrauterine posture, oligohydramnios leading to contractures, and intrinsic abnormalities of the feet.
c. Initially the deformity may be corrected by splinting or serial cast correction. In more severe cases, surgical correction with release of contracted structures may be necessary.

33.
a. Hypertrophic calf muscles.
b. Duchenne muscular dystrophy. Becker's muscular dystrophy has a similar appearance at a later age but has a milder course.
c. Gower sign on rising from the floor, proximal weakness including shoulder girdle, increasing weakness and atrophy,

cardiomyopathy, and variable educational and speech delay.

d. Measurement of serum creatinine phosphokinase, electromyography, muscle biopsy showing absent or abnormal dystrophin and ultrasound of the muscles. The gene defect can now be identified.

e. This is an X-linked recessive condition. The gene defect has been identified at Xp21, the dystrophin gene, which codes for dystrophin, a 400 kDa protein. Dystrophin gene deletion is present in 60% of cases. Mutations in the same gene cause milder Becker's muscular dystrophy.

34.
a. Incontinentia pigmenti—pigmented whorls that start as blisters and do not cross the midline.

b. Apathy, feeding difficulties, failure to thrive, epilepsy and cerebral palsy.

c. X-linked dominant. The majority of males die in utero.

35.
a. Umbilical hernia with herniation of the bowel through a defect at the base of the umbilicus, often associated with diastasis recti. It is especially common in low birth weight and black babies.

b. Most umbilical hernias resolve within the first year of life, so no treatment is required. Surgery is not advised unless the hernia persists to the age of 3–5 years.

36.
a. Herpes simplex stomatitis.

b. Symptomatic treatment with analgesia, rehydration and mouth care. Superadded infection should be treated. Anecdotally, acyclovir may give symptomatic relief but does not alter the course of the disease.

c. Full recovery is usual, but herpes simplex is a latent virus and can recur.

37.
a. This X-ray shows marked cavitation in the left upper lobe and extensive consolidation throughout the left lung consistent with pulmonary tuberculosis (TB).

b. The Mantoux skin test (an intradermal injection on the volar aspect of the arm of purified tuberculous antigen) will usually be positive. The ultimate diagnosis relies on identifying the organism *Mycobacterium tuberculosis* by culture of the sputum.

c. The child should be treated with 6–9 months of combination antituberculous therapy. Contacts should be traced and assessed for disease by chest X-ray and Heaf test. Some contacts may require vaccination with BCG, or chemoprophylaxis with antituberculous therapy.

38.
a. Sturge–Weber syndrome—vascular naevus of the face with a similar angiomatous malformation involving the meninges on the ipsilateral side of the brain.
b. Ophthalmic complications are common and include congenital glaucoma, buphthalmos, telangiectasia of the conjunctiva, and varicosities of retinal vessels.
c. Epilepsy (50–90% of patients), learning difficulties, hemianopia, hemiparesis and subarachnoid haemorrhage.
d. Skull X-ray would reveal linear zones of calcification following contours of gyri appearing as 'double tramlines'. Computed tomography (CT) may reveal calcification, cortical atrophy and abnormalities of the choroid plexus and deep venous system. Magnetic resonance imaging (MRI) correlates with CT scans but does not appear to improve the sensitivity in diagnosis. Angiography may demonstrate abnormalities in cortical veins.
e. There is no evidence that Sturge–Weber syndrome is an inherited disorder. The most probable cause is a new mutation occurring sporadically.

39.
a. Ectopia vesicae—a defect ranging from small cutaneous fistula in the abdominal wall to complete exstrophy of the cloaca, involving exposure of the entire hindgut and bladder.
b. This defect needs extensive surgical repair, and continence is rarely achieved.

40.
a. Distended loops of small bowel and pathognomonic rings of intramural gas in the bowel wall.
b. Necrotising enterocolitis (NEC).
c. Oedema and thickening of the bowel wall, gas in the portal vein, perforation of the bowel with free air in the peritoneal cavity which may accumulate centrally or under the diaphragm, or outline of the falciform ligament in a supine radiograph. Since an erect film can rarely be performed, a lateral decubitus view is often helpful to demonstrate free gas.

41.
a. Extended breech posture. Note the positional talipes.
b. Oedema to the gonads, traumatic delivery and a risk of dislocation of the hips if extended breech presentation.
c. These children should have their hips carefully examined, and should be referred for ultrasound of the hip joint to exclude congenital hip dysplasia.

42.
a. Ectodermal dysplasia.
b. Fine, scanty hair, absent sweat glands, sparse hair growth, peg- or cone-shaped teeth, and depressed nasal bridge.

Patients suffer from chronic upper respiratory tract infections due to an absence of mucous glands.

c. Either X-linked or autosomal recessive.

43.
a. Haemangioma involving the lower lip, chin and oropharynx.
b. The lesion may cause obstruction of the airway. Vascular lesions, which by virtue of their size and site compromise vital structures such as the airway or eyes, may occasionally need emergency treatment with oral steroids.

44.
a. Sebaceous naevus—an uncommon, small, congenital lesion usually found on the scalp or around the hairline. They appear as a hairless, smooth, yellow waxy plaque.
b. Malignant transformation is not uncommon in these lesions and therefore excision is advised in adolescence. They are very rarely associated with convulsions, mental retardation and other abnormalities.

45.
a. Cornelia de Lange syndrome. The infant has anteverted nostrils, thin lips, carp mouth, hirsuitism, bushy eyebrows and long curly eyelashes.
b. Microcephaly, low birth weight, short stature, small hands, severe developmental delay, hypertonicity at birth, growling cry and hypoplastic nipples.
c. Some children with Cornelia de Lange syndrome have chromosomal abnormalities, but these are not consistently confined to one chromosome. Usually sporadic.

46.
a. The abdominal X-ray shows widespread radio-opaque speckling throughout the abdomen, probably within the bowel (A). The X-ray of the femur and upper tibia shows dense lines of opacification in the metaphyses of the long bones (B).
b. Lead poisoning with evidence of acute ingestion (speckling in the bowel) and chronic deposition in the bones.
c. Assay blood for serum lead levels. Investigate the household for sources of environmental lead, e.g. lead-containing toys, old painted surfaces decorated before lead was removed from paint and cooking pots containing lead.

47.
a. Trisomy 13—Patau syndrome.
b. Cleft lip and palate, microcephaly, microphthalmia, sloping forehead, capillary haemangiomas, congenital heart disease (ventricular septal defects, persistent ductus arteriosus, atrial septal defects), clinodactyly, polydactyly, hypoplastic nails, severe developmental and growth delay, renal and haematological anomalies. Other abnormalities include undescended testes in boys.

c. Due to the multiple and severe malformations associated with this condition, up to 90% of cases die in the first few months. The few survivors are severely disabled.

48.
a. Coarse facial features of congenital hypothyroidism.
b. Lethargy and poor feeding, mottled and dry skin, large tongue, hoarse cry, constipation, abdominal distension, prolonged jaundice, oedema, umbilical hernia and hypothermia.
c. Urgent T_4 should be performed to confirm the diagnosis. The finding of a high TSH level suggests a primary thyroid disorder such as thyroid gland dysgenesis or an inborn error of hormone synthesis. A low T_4 and low TSH would fit with hypothalamic or pituitary hypothyroidism. Technetium-99m isotope scan and thyroid ultrasound are indicated to identify the position of the thyroid gland.
d. Replacement therapy with L-thyroxine $100\mu g/m^2$ per day should be started as soon as the diagnosis is confirmed.
e. Despite early treatment, a significant proportion of children with congenital hypothyroidism have learning difficulties and ataxia.

49.
a. Twin to twin transfusion (fetal transfusion syndrome).
b. Monozygotic twins. This condition is very rare in dizygotic twins.
c. The smaller, paler baby on the right is the donor and may suffer from oligohydramonios, anaemia, hypovolaemia and hypoglycaemia. The larger plethoric recipient on the left is at risk of polyhydramnios, polycythaemia, hypervolaemia, cardiac failure and convulsions.

50.
a. The majority of cells on this film are blasts; the most likely diagnosis is acute lymphoblastic leukaemia (ALL). Further immunophenotyping is essential to confirm the diagnosis of ALL.
b. Good prognostic features in ALL are:
   - age 2–5 years
   - white blood count $< 20 \times 10^9/l$
   - common ALL immunophenotype.
   Poor prognostic features in ALL are:
   - age < 1 year
   - white blood count $> 50 \times 10^9/l$
   - B cell type
   - CNS disease at diagnosis
   - Philadelphia chromosome positive ALL.
c. Anaemia, lethargy, bone pain and easy bruising or bleeding

are common at presentation. Increased susceptibility to infection may predate the diagnosis and continue throughout the treatment period.

d. Combinations of anti-leukaemic chemotherapeutic agents and radiotherapy form the basis of all therapeutic regimens. A dramatic improvement in survival rates has been achieved in the UK since treatment has been carefully planned as part of progressive randomised trials (e.g. UKALL trials). Over 95% of children achieve remission within the first 4 weeks and cyclical therapy continues for at least 2 years. The cure rate at 5 years is approximately 75%. Bone marrow transplantation may be considered for less common forms of childhood leukaemia (e.g. acute myeloid leukaemia) or in ALL with poor risk factors.

51.
a. Giant congenital pigmented naevus (bathing trunk distribution).

b. The risk of malignant transformation exists and may be as high as 40%. The risk correlates with the size of the lesion. Most undergo malignant change before puberty. In some cases, congenital melanoma may arise in giant congenital pigmented naevus from birth.

c. This child has had dermabrasion of the giant congenital pigmented naevus. Dermabrasion will improve the appearance and may remove superficial naevus cells but is unable to alleviate the risk of malignant change. Although complete excision would alleviate the risk of malignant transformation, it may not be possible if there is involvement of vital structures or if a large area is involved. Such surgery requires multiple procedures, skin grafting and blood transfusions to replace the blood loss which is often considerable.

52.
a. Lichen sclerosis et atrophicus. The differential diagnosis includes vulval psoriasis and child sexual abuse.

b. Corticosteroid cream or topical oestrogen. The condition tends to resolve at menarche.

53.
a. Bilateral colobomata of the iris. A coloboma is a defect in which part of one, or a number, of the structures of the eye are missing.

b. A coloboma is frequently an isolated finding but may be associated with abnormal ocular development and embryogenesis. If extensive, it may involve the retina and optic nerve, which will result in visual impairment. Eyelids may be affected and the whole eye may be smaller than normal. Colobomata may be associated with chromosomal syndromes, especially trisomy 13, triploidy and CHARGE syndrome.

54.
a. Imperforate hymen or a paravaginal cyst. In the latter case, it is possible to pass a probe into the vagina alongside the cyst.
b. The imperforate hymen may result in a hydrocolpus, whereby the vagina and, less frequently, the uterus and fallopian tubes become distended with mucinous secretion from fetal and vaginal glands. This may result in an abdominal mass and acute urinary retention in the newborn. Paravaginal cysts, although often quite large, rupture spontaneously.

55.
a. Chorioretinitis.
b. Congenital toxoplasmosis, congenital cytomegalovirus, tuberculosis, sarcoidosis or toxocara infestation.
c. It may lead to glaucoma or retinal detachment.

56.
a. Bilateral inguinal hernia.
b. Urgent surgical intervention is necessary for an incarcerated inguinal hernia to prevent bowel necrosis. Reducible hernias should also be repaired electively as soon as possible, as a high proportion of hernias in infancy develop strangulation.

57.
a. The X-ray shows marked cardiomegaly, but there are no radiological signs of pulmonary plethora or oligaemia.
b. Cardiomyopathy due to storage disease, e.g. Pompe (type 2 glycogen storage disease) or viral infection are the most likely diagnoses. A pericardial effusion may have a similar appearance on chest X-ray. Cardiomegaly due to cardiac failure is unlikely in the absence of pulmonary plethora.
c. An electrocardiogram may demonstrate ventricular hypertrophy and exclude conduction defects and arrythmias. Echocardiogram will identify a cardiomyopathy (ventricular septal hypertrophy or poor contractility), pericardial effusion or other structural abnormalities of the heart. The diagnosis of Pompe disease can be confirmed by finding vacuolated lymphocytes in the peripheral blood.

58.
a. Cryptorchidism (undescended or ectopic testes) with scrotal hypoplasia. The majority of undescended testes lie in the inguinal canal. Other sites include intra-abdominal, suprapubic, femoral or perineal. Crytorchidism is bilateral in one-third of cases.
b. If the testes are palpable in the inguinal canal then orchidopexy should be carried out by age 2 years. If the

testes are impalpable then every attempt should be made to locate them. Ultrasonography, magnetic resonance scanning or laparoscopy may be needed to locate the testes. If the testes are intra-abdominal then microvascular orchidopexy will be required. If there is evidence of a spermatic cord without testes, or if the spermatic cord and testes are both absent, then the parents should be counselled and hormone replacement and a testicular prosthesis may be required. Bilateral cryptorchidism with hypospadius requires urgent investigation.

c. If orchidopexy is performed for undescended testes before the age of 2 years then they remain capable of spermatogenesis. After puberty, the intra-abdominal testis should be removed, as it will be incapable of spermatogenesis and the risk of malignancy is much greater than that of a normal testis. Other complications include indirect inguinal hernias and torsion of cryptorchid testis.

59.

a. Posterior fractures of 6, 7, and 8 left ribs posteriorly with callus formation.

b. Posterior rib fractures in infancy are usually the result of a squeezing injury to the thoracic cage and are almost pathognomonic of non-accidental injury. Finger bruises may also be seen on the thorax if the injury is recent. The presence of callus indicates that the injury is more than 72 hours old. In preterm infants, osteopenia of prematurity or copper deficiency may also result in pathological fractures with minor trauma, but these conditions are extremely rare with appropriate nutritional supplementation.

c. A skeletal survey and/or isotope bone scan should be performed to ascertain whether there are multiple fractures. Injuries of varying age are highly suspicious of non-accidental injury. The social circumstances of the family should be carefully assessed when a young infant is injured. Blood should be taken to exclude neonatal rickets, and also copper deficiency in a very preterm infant.

60.

a. • Overfeeding
   • Prader–Willi syndrome
   • Beckwith–Weidemann syndrome
   • Sotos syndrome
   • Laurence–Moon–Biedl syndrome.

b. • Hypotonia, cryptorchidism, small hands and feet suggest Prader–Willi.
   • Macrosomia, omphalocele, macroglossia and ear creases suggest Beckwith–Wiedemann syndrome.

- Macrocephaly, large hands and feet suggest Sotos syndrome.
- Polydactyly and retinal pigmentation suggest Laurence–Moon–Biedl syndrome.

61.

a. Hirschprung's disease, meconium ileus, or a distal intestinal obstruction due to stenosis or webs. A meconium plug can cause obstruction in the early neonatal period.

b. Hirschprung's disease is diagnosed by rectal biopsy, looking for absent ganglion cells in submucosa, and nerve fibres with increased acetylcholinesterase. Meconium ileus can be suspected on a plain abdominal X-ray if there is marked distension of bowel or a 'snowstorm' appearance in the abdomen due to air within viscid meconium. Gastrointestinal perforation and meconium peritonitis may lead to intra-abdominal calcification. Other causes of intestinal obstruction can be confirmed by contrast studies.

c. The treatment depends on the underlying pathology. Hirschprung's disease requires colostomy at the most distal portion of normal colon. A definitive pull-through procedure is performed at a later date. Meconium ileus may be managed by the administration of hyperosmolar and mucolytic agents. If these fail, or if there is an associated atresia, then surgical resection and anastomosis will be required. Distal stenosis, atresias or webs required surgical correction.

62.

a. Spherocytosis—there are multiple small densely staining spherocytes. These are large blue young red cells which are polychromatic and would be reticulocytes on appropriate staining.

b. Hyperbilirubinaemia or prolonged neonatal jaundice is common in congenital spherocytosis. ABO incompatibility may also cause similar clinical and haematological features in the newborn. The anaemia of congenital spherocytosis is variable in severity and can present at any age. Fluctuating jaundice, splenomegaly and gallstones may eventually occur.

c. There should be careful follow-up and monitoring of the anaemia and growth throughout childhood. Splenectomy is not usually indicated unless there is severe anaemia needing repeated blood transfusions, hypersplenism, gallstones or failure to thrive. Other family members should also be investigated for congenital spherocytosis, as it is often an autosomal dominant condition.

63.

a. Free gas under the diaphragm. This child had intestinal obstruction, hence the dilated loops of bowel.

b. This occurs after gastrointestinal perforation and there would be signs of peritonitis, including abdominal tenderness, guarding, rebound, bile-stained vomiting and absent bowel sounds. Less commonly, free gas can occur after laparoscopy or laparotomy.

64.
a. Palatal petechiae, hirsuitism and facial striae.
b. Aplastic anaemia. The palatal petechiae are secondary to thrombocytopenia, and the hirsuitism and facial striae are due to corticosteroid and cyclosporin therapy.
c. Supportive therapy includes blood and platelet transfusions, immunosuppression with corticosteroids, cyclosporin and the use of antithymocyte globulin or antilymphocyte globulin or androgens. Aggressive broad-spectrum antimicrobials are required for periods of sepsis. Definitive therapy with matched bone marrow transplant or stem cells from umbilical blood may be curative and is now the preferred treatment.

65.
a. Hypertrophy of the right limb.
b. Hypertrophy of the limb is associated with Klippel–Trenaunay–Weber, Beckwith–Wiedemann syndrome, Wilms tumour, congenital hemihypertrophy, haemangioma, hypomelanosis of Ito and neurofibromatosis.
c. Wilms tumour is found in 1 in 30 patients who have isolated hemihypertrophy. Renal ultrasound should be performed periodically.

66.
a. Brushfield spots found in 75% of children with Down syndrome.
b. Epicanthic folds, small midface, brachycephaly, flat occiput, Brushfield spots, upward slanting palpebral fissures, prominent tongue and small mouth, short broad hands, single palmar crease, short stature, developmental delay, hypotonia, delayed closure of fontanelle, laxity of atlantoaxial articulation, increased incidence of hypothyroidism, Hirschprung's disease, leukaemia and Alzheimer disease.
c. Forty per cent of infants with Down syndrome have congenital heart disease. The commonest lesions are atrioventricular canal defect or ventricular septal defect. Without surgery, these lesions may lead to pulmonary hypertension. Other conditions include tetralogy of Fallot or a patent ductus arteriosus.

67.
a. Congenital pigmented naevus.
b. Naevi overlying the head may be associated with leptomeningeal melanocytosis, which may result in hydrocephalus, seizures and learning difficulties. Magnetic resonance imaging may identify involvement of the central

nervous system. These lesions carry a significant lifetime risk of malignant melanoma, but probably less so than the giant congenital pigmented naevi.

c. With a risk of malignant change, some authorities recommend early surgical excision, but this may prove difficult if there is involvement of fascia or meninges. Alternatives are dermabrasion, split thickness excisions or serial examinations. Leptomeningeal melanoma has been reported to occur despite excision of these lesions.

68.

a. Strawberry naevus (capillary haemangioma)—bright red protuberant vascular lesions, appearing in the first 2 months of age. This photograph demonstrates the typical appearance of a resolving naevus.

b. The majority increase in size rapidly during the first year of life. They spontaneously regress over subsequent years, leaving only a flat pale depigmented area.

c. Ten per cent of patients are left with small cosmetic defect. The naevus may ulcerate and develop secondary infection. They may encroach on vital organs, e.g. eyes and airway, and massive lesions can lead to a consumption thrombocytopenia — Kasabach–Merritt syndrome. Where there is pressure on a vital organ or severe bleeding, steroids may be helpful. Otherwise, no treatment is required.

69.

a. Left Erb's palsy—the left arm is held loosely at the side of the thorax, internally rotated and extended at the elbow; the forearm is pronated and there is flexion of the wrist (waiter's tip position). This condition may follow the traumatic delivery of a large for dates baby.

b. Stretching or tearing of the upper brachial plexus (C5–6) with denervation of the deltoid, supraspinatus biceps and brachioradialis.

c. Most neurological recovery occurs within the first few months. Fewer than 20% have permanent neurological deficit. If the condition does not improve by 6 weeks, surgical exploration of the brachial plexus may be required. Some affected infants may have aplasia of the brachial plexus.

70.

a. Infant of a diabetic mother or Beckwith–Weidemann syndrome.

b. Infants of diabetic mothers are at increased risk of birth injury, hypoglycaemia, respiratory distress, jaundice, polycythaemia, hypocalcaemia, poor sucking, and cardiomyopathy due to septal hypertrophy. They have a higher incidence of neural tube defects, ventricular septal defects, transposition of great vessels, coarctation of the aorta, vertebral anomalies, sacral agenesis, renal vein thrombosis and anorectal anomalies. Beckwith–Weidemann syndrome is associated with omphalocele, macrosomia and macroglossia, facial naevus flammus and a characteristic earlobe crease.

71.
a. Hypochromic, microcytic red cells of varying size (anisocytosis) and cigar-shaped red cells.
b. Iron deficiency anaemia or β-thalassaemia trait. Red cell indices may help to differentiate between these conditions. Cigar-shaped cells are a feature of iron deficiency, but are not seen in β-thalassaemia.
c. Detailed dietary history, history of gastrointestinal blood loss, ethnic background and family history of haemoglobinopathy.
d. Iron studies, e.g. serum ferritin and total iron binding capacity, are often performed but are rarely diagnostic. If the history is suggestive of poor dietary intake of iron, a rising haemoglobin in response to iron therapy is the best confirmation of the diagnosis of iron deficiency anaemia. Haemoglobin electrophoresis, including HbA_2 quantification to exclude β-thalassaemia trait, should be performed when the child is iron replete.

72.
a. Chickenpox—varicella zoster infection. This is a highly contagious infection in childhood, with >90% of children affected by age 10 years. Fever, malaise and anorexia may occur in the 24 hours preceding the rash. The rash is characteristic with vesicles on an erythematous base, which appear in crops, ulcerate, crust and heal over 10–14 days.
b. The incubation period is generally 14–16 days, with a range of 11–20 days. The period of infectivity begins 2 days before the onset of the rash and ends when all the lesions are crusted.
c. Chickenpox is usually a mild disease, but complications are common. They include:
   - secondary infection of skin lesions by streptococci or staphylococci
   - thrombocytopenia and haemorrhagic lesions
   - cerebellar ataxia, postinfectious encephalitis, Guillain–Barré
   - pneumonia, myocarditis, hepatitis
   - Reye syndrome in association with aspirin ingestion.
   - varicella is a serious disease in neonates, in the first week after birth, during pregnancy and in immunosuppressed individuals including those on corticosteroid therapy.

73.
a. Superior vena cava obstruction with distended neck veins.
b. A lymphoma, the commonest malignancy in teenagers. Massive lymphadenopathy from other conditions such as tuberculosis may also cause this syndrome.
c. Airway obstruction. If steroid therapy is administered, the patient is at risk from 'tumour lysis syndrome'. Chemotherapy administered to patients with large tumours may result in massive cell lysis, leading to hypocalcaemia, hyperkalaemia, hyperuricaemia and hyperphosphataemia. This can be avoided by pretreatment hydration and allopurinol administration (a xanthine oxidase inhibitor).

74.
a. This photograph shows signs of respiratory distress with sternal and subcostal recession. This gives the appearance of pectus excavatum. This breathing pattern may occur with upper airway obstruction such as tonsillar swelling, acute laryngotracheobronchitis or inhaled foreign body, or lower airway disease such as bronchospasm due to asthma.
b. Treatment should be directed towards the cause. Foreign bodies should be removed and respiratory distress from acute laryngotracheobronchitis may be relieved by adrenaline nebulisers. Bronchospasm will improve with the use of nebulised bronchodilators. Massive tonsillar hypertrophy may necessitate steroid therapy and antibiotics.

75.
a. Meningococcal septicaemia.
b. Initially, the child will need resuscitation, venous access, high-dose intravenous third-generation cephalosporin or penicillin, and large volumes of colloid. Subsequent management will involve transfer to intensive care for ventilation, inotrope therapy for myocardial dysfunction, correction of electrolyte disturbance and acidosis, prevention of raised intracranial pressure in the presence of meningitis, management of acute respiratory distress syndrome (ARDS) and treatment of coagulopathy.
c. Meningococcal septicaemia carries a mortality greater than 30%. This figure is reduced to less than 20% in the presence of meningitis.
d. Prophylactic rifampicin should be administered to close family contacts.

76.
a. Ichthyosis—an inherited skin condition with abnormal keratinisation characterised by visible scaling.
b. Milder forms may be treated with simple emollients or mild keratolytics such as salicylic acid in aqueous cream. In the more severe form, careful nursing and medical care are

required to avoid secondary infection and to compensate for losses of water, electrolytes and protein.

c. Many collodion infants develop ichthyotic skin changes in childhood. There is an increased incidence of atopy.

77.
a. Rickets—note the thickening of the wrist bones.
b. Poor linear growth, bowing of legs, thickening at wrists and knees, prominence of the costochondral junctions, frontal skull bossing, hypotonia and delayed closure of the anterior fontanelle.
c. A detailed dietary history must be obtained, as well as serum calcium, serum phosphate, serum alkaline phosphatase and vitamin D levels. Wrist X-rays may show a wide growth plate, cupped metaphysis, diminished calcification and a secondary centre of ossification in the epiphysis.
d. Vitamin D supplementation. The dose depends on the underlying cause.

78.
a. Diaphragmatic hernia with herniation of the bowel through a defect in the left side of the diaphragm, resulting in mediastinal shift. The apex beat will be displaced towards the right and there will be reduced breath sounds in the left lung on auscultation of the chest. The heart sounds will most easily be heard in the right hemithorax. The abdomen may be scaphoid in appearance. The diagnosis is often made on antenatal ultrasound.
b. Emergency resuscitation with intubation and ventilation. Continuous drainage of gas from the stomach using a large bore nasogastric tube is mandatory. Management of persistent pulmonary hypertension (PPHT) using prostacyclin, high-frequency oscillation or nitric oxide is often necessary before definitive surgery is performed. It is usual to delay surgery until the newborn is stable.
c. Survival has improved in recent years with pre-operative stabilisation and management of PPHT, but is still only 60–70% because of underlying pulmonary hypoplasia in a high proportion of cases with a large hernia.

79.
a. The skin appearance could be due to a healing eschar. However the wrist X-ray demonstrates extensive subcutaneous calcification of the soft tissue.
b. This resulted from extravasated intravenous feed containing calcium.

80.
a. Papilloedema shown by blurring of the optic disc, distortion of blood vessels, and nerve fibre layer haemorrhages around the disc.

b. At this age and with this history, the most likely diagnosis is an intracranial tumour. Other causes of papilloedema include intracranial haemorrhage, hypertension, benign intracranial hypertension and cerebral oedema.

81.
a. There is a large proportion of sickle cells present. Other features that may be present in sickle cell disease but which are not shown on this film include target cells and polychromasia.

b. Sickle cell disease.

c. A sickle solubility screening test will be positive. Haemoglobin electrophoresis confirms the presence of the individual types of haemoglobin. Homozygous sickle cell disease is the most common diagnosis, with mainly HbS and absent HbA. HbSC and Hb S thalassaemia may also present with similar clinical features and peripheral blood film.

d. Symptoms of sickle cell disease rarely present before the age of 6 months. Painful crises affecting the long bones, joints and abdomen, often associated with a fever, are the most common symptoms. Infection, dehydration and acidosis are all potential precipitating factors. In younger children, infarction with painful swelling of the short bones of the hands and feet causes a characteristic 'hand–foot syndrome' (dactylitis). Infarction may be difficult to distinguish from osteomyelitis in the early stages and children with sickle cell disease are susceptible to *Salmonella* and *Haemophilus influenzae* osteomyelitis. Aplastic crises may occur with *Parvovirus*.

e. The family must be educated to detect and treat acutely painful crises early with adequate hydration and analgesia. Prophylactic penicillin should be given. Pneumovax and *Haemophilus influenzae* type B immunisation is indicated at the appropriate age. Antenatal diagnosis can also be offered in subsequent pregnancies.

82.
a. Orbital cellulitis (right eye)—bacterial infection of the orbit, usually arising from the ethmoid sinus in older patients or from local infection in infants. The most common causative organisms are *Streptococcus*, *Staphylococcus* and *Haemophilus influenzae*. The incidence of orbital cellulitis due to the latter has fallen since the introduction of *Haemophilus influenzae* type B (Hib) vaccination.

b. Systemic spread of the organism may result in bacteraemia. Local spread can lead to abscess formation in the orbit, resulting in ophthalmoplegia, vision loss and proptosis, or a cavernous sinus thrombosis leading to headache, nuchal rigidity and cranial nerve palsy.

c. Throat swab, blood cultures and full blood count. Lumbar puncture should be considered.

d. Broad-spectrum intravenous antibiotics and analgesia, and monitor for complications.

83.

a. Cutis aplasia—congenital absence of skin on the scalp.

b. This may be an isolated defect but is commonly associated with trisomy 13, where there may be defects in the bones of the scalp.

c. Karyotype to exclude trisomy 13.

d. The defect heals by granulation but may lead to scar formation and contraction. A permanent bald patch may be left on the scalp.

84.

a. Air enema.

b. Intussusception—the obstruction is evident in the proximal transverse colon, with cupping of the air at the head of the intussusception. Intussusception is most often ileocolic and is therefore found in the right upper quadrant.

c. Plain abdominal X-ray is rarely diagnostic but may show absence of gas in the area of the intussusception. Ultrasound may identify the mass. Barium or air enema will demonstrate the filling defect, and barium may be seen trapped around the invaginating intestine. Air enema is now preferred and may be used under pressure to reduce the intussusception.

d. Reduction of the intussusception is an emergency procedure to be performed immediately after diagnosis. Often, reduction occurs at the time of the diagnostic enema if the history is short. Appropriate analgesia should be given and intravenous administration of colloid is often necessary. If the history is greater than 48 hours, or if there is evidence of peritonitis, laparotomy and manual operative reduction are indicated because of the risk of perforation.

85.

a. This coronal view shows bilateral intraventricular haemorrhage (IVH) and a grade IV left-sided periventricular or intracerebral haemorrhage (PVH).

b. IVH occurs in 10–40% of preterm infants less than 33 weeks gestation. It is more common in infants who have had adverse antenatal or intrapartum events affecting cerebral blood flow and in those who have had severe respiratory distress after birth. IVH is usually asymptomatic, but intracerebral or periventricular haemorrhage is often associated with neonatal convulsions. Rapidly progressive posthaemorrhagic hydrocephalus may cause apnoea.

c. Serial cranial ultrasonography is important in the first 2 weeks of life to document the extent of haemorrhagic lesions.

Grade I and II IVH are not associated with any increased long-term risk. The long-term prognosis correlates well with the presence or absence of periventricular leukomalcia (PVL) at 6 weeks of age. Some infarcted areas may develop into a porencephalic cyst of variable long-term significance depending on the site of the lesion.

86.
a. Infantile seborrhoeic dermatitis, a common acute erythematous scaly eruption affecting the scalp or napkin area.
b. Bland emollient, olive oil, topical 0.5% or 1% hydrocortisone alone or in combination with antifungal, or topical salicylate for thick scaling.
c. The condition is self-limiting within the first year of life.

87.
a. The differential diagnosis is either an occipital meningocele (a cystic swelling arising through a skull bone defect and containing only cerebrospinal fluid) or an occipital encephalocele with abnormal brain tissue in the sac. The latter may be associated with myelomeningocele, microcephalus, hydrocephalus and cleft palate.
b. Approximately half of the infants who require surgery for an occipital meningocele are neurologically normal. The outcome for occipital encephalocele is much worse, as the rest of the brain is often grossly abnormal and the vast majority have severe neurological impairment.

88.
a. Goitre (enlarged thyroid).
b. Goitre plus hyperthyroidism occurs in Graves' disease, early Hashimoto's thyroiditis or thyroid tumours.
c. The symptoms of hyperthyroidism may be treated with propranolol. Definitive treatment is with carbimazole or propylthiouracil. Thyroidectomy may be indicated.

89.
a. Suppurative cervical adenitis.
b. It arises secondary to upper respiratory tract infections, e.g. streptococcal sore throat or staphylococcal infection. Other causes of cervical lymphadenopathy include:
   - tonsillitis or pharyngitis
   - local infection with Epstein–Barr virus, tuberculosis, or atypical mycobacterium
   - malignancy, e.g. lymphoma
   - part of a generalised lymphadenopathy, e.g. viral illnesses such as Epstein–Barr virus, malignancy, toxoplasmosis, autoimmune disease.
c. Full blood count and film, Monospot for Epstein–Barr virus, ESR, chest X-ray, serum for viral titres, blood cultures, and throat swab for microbiology and viral culture.

d. If a bacterial cause is isolated, appropriate antibiotics should be administered. If the lymphadenopathy enlarges and becomes fluctuant with pus, surgical drainage may be indicated.

90.
a. Ambiguous genitalia where the gender cannot be determined by clinical examination alone. In this case, there was virilisation with fused labia and cliteromegaly due to congenital adrenal hyperplasia in a female infant.
b. It is important to determine if the disorder represents virilisation of a female infant (androgen excess), or a male infant with severe hypospadias and bilateral cryptorchidism. Gonads that are evident on palpation are usually testes, and absence of female internal genitalia on pelvic ultrasound implies underdevelopment of the male. This can be confirmed by karyotype. Most virilised females have congenital adrenal hyperplasia due to 21-hydroxylase deficiency. This can be confirmed by finding an elevated plasma 17-hydroxyprogesterone after the first few days of life. In addition, there will be an abnormal urinary steroid profile. Serum electrolytes and plasma renin should be determined. The plasma renin will be elevated with hyponatraemia and hyperkalaemia if the infant is salt-losing in an adrenal crisis.
c. This infant is likely to develop adrenal crisis with vomiting and hyponatraemia. She may require intravenous glucose, saline and hydrocortisone as part of the initial resuscitation. The infant will require lifelong physiological replacement of glucocorticoid (hydrocortisone), and mineralocorticoid (fludrocortisone) if salt-losing. Assigning gender must be carefully considered after determining the nature of the hormonal defect and the feasibility of genital reconstruction. Surgical repair must be carefully planned. Dysgenetic gonads should be removed because of the risk of malignant change.

91.
a. Mucosal neuromas.
b. Part of multiple endocrine neoplasia (MEN) type 2B. Associated with phaeochromocytoma, marfanoid appearance and medullary thyroid carcinoma. Also associated with constipation secondary to hyperganglionosis.
c. Investigate for medullary thyroid carcinoma by basal measurement of serum calcitonin and after provocation by pentagastrin; 24 hour collection for urinary catecholamines. Genetic studies are available—the MEN2 locus is linked to chromosome 10.
d. There is a 100% risk of aggressive medullary thyroid carcinoma in children born with MEN2B.
e. All affected children should be referred for thyroidectomy.

92.
a. Bilateral cleft lip and palate.
b. Most lesions are isolated defects. Cleft palate may be part of a syndrome, e.g. Pierre Robin sequence, trisomy 13. Other malformations occur in 15% of cases.
c. Initial feeding difficulties and poor weight gain, middle ear infection, aspiration pneumonia, speech difficulty and nasal voice, and orthodontic problems.
d. A multidisciplinary approach is required, involving surgeons, speech therapy, orthodontic and hearing assessment. Repair of the lip is usually within 3 months of birth, and the palate by 6 months before vocalisation develops. In the school age child, alveolar bone grafting may be required. Children should be monitored for serous otitis media, reading difficulties and psychological problems. In adolescence, some patients require surgical treatment for midface retrusion and rhinoplasty.

93.
a. Gastric aspirate containing epithelial debris and Gram-positive cocci in chains typical of group B streptococci.
b. Prematurity, prolonged rupture of membranes >24 hours, maternal pyrexia and intrapartum sepsis, e.g. amnionitis.
c. Only 1% of infants who are colonised with group B streptococci develop invasive disease. The earliest clinical sign is persistent tachypnoea >60 breaths/min within the first 24 hours of life. Apnoea, poor feeding and respiratory distress related to pneumonia are late manifestations of the fulminating septicaemia caused by group B streptococcus. The onset of symptoms in meningitis caused by this organism at a later age is usually more insidious.

94.
a. Hydrops fetalis—generalised oedema, ascites and pleural effusions; some cases have hepatosplenomegaly.
b. Many cases are secondary to severe fetal anaemia, e.g. rhesus disease, α-thalassaemia or intrauterine infection with parvovirus resulting in severe aplastic anaemia. Other causes include congenital infections, e.g. toxoplasma, cytomegalovirus, cardiac failure and supraventricular tachycardias, hypoproteinaemia, twin to twin transfusion or a placental angioma. Many cases are idiopathic.
c. Affected babies frequently need intubation at the delivery. If large pleural effusions are present, these may need to be drained urgently. If there is severe anaemia, early exchange transfusion and ventilatory support are required. Arrhythmias should be corrected with drugs or defibrillation.

95.

a. (A) shows café au lait macules. (B) demonstrates neurofibromata and the surgical scar from Harrington Rod insertion for scoliosis.

b. Neurofibromatosis type 1.

c. In order to make the diagnosis, the individual must have two or more of the following criteria:
   - six or more café au lait macules, ≥5 mm in prepubertal or ≥15 mm in postpubertal children
   - two or more neurofibromas
   - axillary freckling
   - optic glioma
   - oris hamartomas
   - one osseous lesion
   - a first-degree relative with type 1 neurofibromatosis.

d. Autosomal dominant. There is a 50% risk of transmission; 50% are new mutations. The chromosome defect has been mapped to chromosome 17.

96.

a. Idiopathic scrotal oedema—erythema and swelling of the scrotum, with non-tender testes. This condition is probably an allergic condition, although the precipitating allergen is rarely identified.

b. It is imperative to exclude other causes of the acute scrotum, including torsion of the testis, epididymo-orchitis, torsion of the testicular appendage or incarcerated hernia which may require urgent surgery. These conditions are associated with severe pain and tenderness, whereas idiopathic scrotal oedema usually causes only mild discomfort. Idiopathic scrotal oedema is a self-limiting condition with spontaneous resolution within 48 hours, although antihistamines may relieve the pain and swelling more rapidly.

97.

a. Laurence–Moon–Biedl syndrome, Prader–Willi syndrome, hypothyroidism or simple obesity.

b. Laurence–Moon–Biedl is inherited as an autosomal recessive condition. The inheritance of Prader–Willi syndrome demonstrates *genomic imprinting*, whereby genetic material is expressed differentially depending on whether it is maternal or paternal in origin. If the gene deletion is on the paternally inherited chromosome 15, the child will have Prader–Willi syndrome. Conversely, if the deletion is on the maternally acquired chromosome 15, the clinical expression is that of Angelman syndrome.

c. Laurence–Moon–Biedl syndrome is associated with hypogonadism secondary to gonadotrophin deficiency, retinitis pigmentosa, developmental delay, polydactyly and obesity. Individuals with this disorder also have an increased incidence of hypertension, diabetes mellitus, and renal and cardiac anomalies.

The clinical features of Prader–Willi syndrome are age-dependent. In the neonatal period, infants present with poor feeding and hypotonia. During infancy they fail to thrive, with developmental delay, and then later develop a voracious appetite and become obese, with short stature and delayed secondary sexual development.

Features of hypothyroidism after infancy include poor growth, weight gain and coarse facies, pallor, sinus bradycardia, muscle weakness, cold intolerance and poor school performance.

98.
a. Gallows traction—the legs are strapped and attached to an elevated bar so that the buttocks are lifted off the mattress.
b. It is used for treatment of a fractured femur or reduction of an inguinal hernia.

99.
a. Anencephaly—a severe neural tube defect with failure of fusion of the skull bones and skin, exposing the malformed rudimentary brain. Most cases are diagnosed in the antenatal period by detailed ultrasonography, and termination of pregnancy can then be considered.
b. This condition is incompatible with life. Many infants are stillborn, although a few may survive for some days. Liveborn infants may be suitable donors for heart transplantation for other infants.
c. All pregnant mothers should take folic acid prior to conception and throughout the first trimester to reduce the risk of neural tube defects. If a previous pregnancy has resulted in an infant with a neural tube defect, the mother should be advised to take a higher dose of folic acid in subsequent pregnancies.

100.
a. Thrombocytopenia purpura. In children, this is usually idiopathic.
b. Immunoglobulin concentrations, viral titres for cytomegalovirus, mycoplasma and Epstein–Barr virus.
c. Clinical symptoms or signs that suggest an alternative diagnosis such as leukaemia are indications for bone marrow aspirate. These include pallor, lassitude, pain, limp, lymphadenopathy or hepatosplenomegaly. Abnormal white cells on blood film, failure to remit after 3 weeks, or if treatment with steroids is contemplated are other indications for bone marrow examination.
d. This is controversial. The risk of intracranial haemorrhage

with idiopathic thrombocytopenia is only 1%. Steroid therapy or intravenous immunoglobulin will cause a rise in platelet count slightly faster than would no treatment. However, these measures do not affect the prognosis. Treatment should be considered if there is mucosal bleeding, neurological signs or a history of recent head trauma. Splenectomy may be curative in the small number of children who have prolonged, persistent thrombocytopenia.

e. For the majority of cases, the prognosis is excellent. Chronic thrombocytopenia purpura, defined as thrombocytopenia persisting beyond 6 months, occurs in 10–20% of patients. There are no long-term sequelae other than complications associated with rare serious haemorrhage in the early stages of the disease.

101.

a. The most likely cause is listeria infection, but *Pseudomonas* or *Klebsiella* sepsis may give a similar skin ulceration. Epidermolysis bullosa presents with more extensive blistering. The organism, *Listeria monocytogenes*, may be present in soft unpasteurized cheeses and salads, and is more commonly found in Europe than in the UK. Listeriosis is associated with intrauterine death and neonatal meningitis.

b. The baby will require a full septic work-up, including blood cultures, full blood count, lumbar puncture, chest X-ray and swabs of the skin lesions.

c. The baby will need resuscitation, ventilation and early administration of high-dose broad-spectrum antibiotics. Ampicillin and gentamicin are the preferred antibiotic treatment for listeriosis. With early treatment, survival has improved in recent years.

102.

a. Short webbed neck with asymmetrical position of the scapulae. Although a webbed neck is found in Turner and Noonan syndrome, the abnormal position of the scapulae is not a feature. The diagnosis is a Sprengel deformity.

b. The cause is a developmental anomaly in which there is failure of the scapula to descend from its embryonic position in the neck.

103.

a. Osteogenesis imperfecta, with angular deformities of limbs from previous fractures and chest deformity. Similar chest deformity is seen in Morquio syndrome (mucopolysaccharidosis type IV).

b. Excessive bone fragility resulting in frequent fractures, blue sclerae, conductive hearing loss and low birth weight.

c. This depends on the type: autosomal dominant (commonest non-lethal variant), autosomal recessive (lethal) or heterogenous. Lethal variants probably result from a mutation of genes coding for alpha 1 or 2 chains of type 1 collagen.

104.
a. The pathology specimen shows mucosal oedema and ulceration, pseudopolyps and a sharp demarcation line at the level of the caecum. This is consistent with ulcerative colitis.
b. Ulcerative colitis presents with a history of bloody diarrhoea with mucus, tenesmus and urgency, abdominal pain and lethargy. On examination, the patient may be anaemic, may demonstrate growth failure, and may have extraintestinal manifestations of inflammatory bowel disease such as erythema nodosum or arthropathy.

105.
a. Anal Crohn's disease with anal tags and sinuses. Child sexual abuse should be considered.
b. Abdominal pain, diarrhoea, blood per rectum, weight loss, growth failure, pallor, mouth ulcers, joint pains and fever.
c. Routine full blood count and ESR, and measurement of C-reactive protein. Full assessment will involve a colonoscopy and biopsy, and barium meal and follow-through.
d. Anal Crohn's disease is difficult to treat, but oral metronidazole, oral steroids, oral or intravenous cyclosporin, or a polymeric diet may help.

106.
a. Phocomelia—hypoplasia of the proximal segment of the limb. In some cases the digits may arise from the stump.
b. These infants need to be managed in a centre with special expertise for children with limb deformities. A multidisciplinary approach should be adopted, with input from orthopaedic and plastic surgeons, occupational and physiotherapy, paediatricians and social services.

107.
a. This photograph shows a foot with convexity of the sole and prominent heels, giving the appearance of 'rocker-bottom feet'.
b. Trisomy 18—Edward syndrome.
c. Horseshoe kidneys are found in over 50% of affected babies. Renal problems may not be apparent at birth or may be so severe as to cause early renal failure.

108.
a. This coronal view shows marked bilateral ventriculomegaly with dilatation of both lateral ventricles, including inferior horns and the interventricular foramina. There is a resolving intraventricular clot on the floor of the right ventricle.
b. Posthaemorrhagic hydrocephalus.
c. Transient or self-limiting hydrocephalus with ventriculomegaly but no increased growth velocity of the

occipitofrontal head circumference does not require any specific treatment if the infant is asymptomatic. If there is recurrent apnoea or respiratory depression, or rapidly progressive hydrocephalus, repeated aspiration of the bloodstained cerebrospinal fluid (CSF) by lumbar puncture or ventricular taps may alleviate symptoms. Early shunt procedures are often complicated by blockage associated with the high protein content of the haemorrhagic CSF. Fewer than 10% of infants with intraventricular haemorrhage have progressive posthaemorrhagic hydrocephalus requiring the insertion of a ventriculoperitoneal shunt at a later stage.

109.
a. Meningococcal meningitis seen as Gram-negative cocci, typically occurring in pairs or clumps with adjacent sides flattened.
b. CSF culture may grow *Neisseria meningitidis*. Nasal carriage in the index case or close relative is common. Circulating antigens can be detected in the serum, CSF and urine using counterimmunoelectrophoresis or latex agglutination techniques. These tests are often positive when the microscopy and culture are negative in a child who has already received antibiotics before investigations have been performed.

110.
a. Non-accidental injury (NAI).
b. There are finger tip marks on the spine, bruising to the buttocks and a possible cigarette burn.
c. Late presentation, a history that is inconsistent with the examination, previous injuries, or concerns from the social services.

111.
a. Napkin dermatitis and candidiasis. This presents as papules, vesicopapules and satellite lesions affecting perineal skin and folds.
b. Topical antifungal agents such as local nystatin and miconazole. Barrier creams, exposure and oral anticandidal therapy may be used in recurrent cases.

112.
a. Erythema nodosum.
b. The commonest causes are tuberculosis and group A streptococcus infection. Other causes to be considered are:
- other bacteria, e.g. *Yersinia*
- viruses, e.g. Epstein–Barr, hepatitis B, measles
- fungi, e.g. histoplasmosis
- malignancies, e.g. Hodgkin's disease, leukaemia
- others, e.g. inflammatory bowel disease, sarcoidosis, oral contraceptive pill, sulphonamides.

No cause is found in many cases.

113.
a. The photograph shows a small midline lesion over the occiput. Note that there is also a capillary naevus (salmon patch) over the neck, which is a common finding in the newborn.
b. Ultrasonography is sometimes helpful to determine if a midline lesion is a small encephalocele or meningocele, but computed tomography or magnetic resonance imaging is often necessary to be certain of the anatomy before surgery.

114.
a. Toxic epidermal necrolysis/scalded skin syndrome—large blister formation, skin erythema, fever and malaise caused by exotoxin-producing staphylococci phage group II. The differential diagnosis includes erythema multiforme and Stevens–Johnson syndrome.
b. Dehydration and shock may occur with extensive lesions.
c. Treatment involves isolation of the patient, fluid replacement and resuscitation, systemic antibiotics and skin care.

115.
a. At 3 days of age, there is widespread periventricular flare in the parasagittal view (A). The ventricle is small and there is no sign of intraventricular haemorrhage. Cystic changes in the area of previous echodensity are developing by 18 days (B), and at 26 days (C) there is extensive cystic periventricular leukomalacia (PVL).
b. Extensive PVL, particularly bilateral, has a poor prognosis, with 80–90% of infants having severe neurodevelopmental impairment, usually cerebral palsy or visual impairment if the lesions are posterior. Unilateral small single cysts, particularly those located in the frontal region, may have a better prognosis.

116.
a. Strabismus; this is demonstrated by an asymmetric light reflex.
b. The patient should be examined for full eye movements, visual acuity to each eye, opththalmoscopy and examination of the orbit. The cover test can be used to determine whether there is a change in fixation and if there is a latent squint.

117.
a. Urticaria—itchy, fluctuating wheals on any part of the body.
b. The cause is often difficult to identify, but the following should be considered: ingestion of drugs and foods such as nuts and food additives, infections, insect bites, or contact with animal dander or plant substances. Children with recurrent urticaria may need investigating to exclude systemic conditions such as malignancy, hyperthyroidism and familial

C1 esterase deficiency. Skin testing for allergens is rarely helpful.

c. Identify and remove the allergen if possible. Administer systemic antihistamines and give prednisolone if severe. Topical relief with calamine lotion may help.

118.

a. Hyperpigmentation of the gingival margins, which is a manifestation of adrenocortical insufficiency. In this age group, the likely cause is Addison's disease. The clinical manifestations depend on the aetiology and age of onset. Older children present with weakness, lassitude and weight loss, and may progress to an adrenal crisis. The increased pigmentation is secondary to excessive production of corticotrophin (ACTH) from the anterior pituitary gland. ACTH has melanocyte-stimulating properties, leading to pigmentation in the hands, face and genitalia.

b. Adrenal crises must be managed with intravenous glucose, saline and hydrocortisone. Once the acute manifestations are under control, the patient will require physiological replacement with hydrocortisone and fludrocortisone. During periods of stress, the dose of hydrocortisone should be increased. Patients with Addison's disease are particularly prone to other autoimmune conditions.

119.

a. Premature pubarche—pubic hair before age 8 years.

b. This may be an isolated finding, in which case a virilising ovarian tumour or congenital adrenal hyperplasia must be excluded. If the development of pubic hair is associated with breast and sexual development and a growth spurt, precocious puberty is the likely diagnosis. This is most commonly idiopathic, but rarely may be secondary to hypothalamic tumours, hydrocephalus, hCG-secreting tumours, ovarian tumours, adrenal tumours or McCune–Albright syndrome.

c. In isolated pubarche, urinary steroids and serum levels of testosterone, 17-hydroxyprogesterone and dehydroepiandrosterone should be measured, and a pelvic ultrasound should be performed. Patients with precocious puberty may require computed tomography or magnetic resonance scanning of the head to exclude a pituitary tumour.

120.

a. Micrognathia. The Pierre Robin sequence is the association of micrognathia and cleft palate with a small retropositioned tongue and glossoptosis. Note the absent auditory meatus in this particular child.

b. The child should be nursed prone and should not sleep on its back. Other abnormalities such as a cleft palate may need treatment. Formal hearing assessment and auditory brain stem-evoked responses should be performed in view of the abnormality of the external ear.

121.
a. Erythema marginatum—an erythematous rash with serpiginous border and central clearing.
b. It frequently results from streptococcal sensitisation.
c. One should look for other features of rheumatic fever. Other major criteria in the Jones system for rheumatic fever are polyarthritis, features of carditis (e.g. new murmur or cardiac failure), chorea or subcutaneous nodules. Minor criteria include fever >38.2°C, arthralgia, leucocytosis, elevated inflammatory markers or prolonged PR interval.

122.
a. Left cataract—opaque mass seen in the pupil.
b. Cataracts may occur as isolated abnormalities. They are also a feature of many syndromes and chromosomal disorders such as Down syndrome. Cataracts may be inherited as an autosomal dominant condition, or associated with intrauterine infection, usually rubella, and metabolic disorders such as galactosaemia. There may be other ocular abnormalities such as microphthalmos.
c. Associated metabolic conditions should be identified and treated as soon as possible. Early referral to an ophthalmologist is imperative as some cataracts require early excision to prevent amblyopia.

123.
a. Poststreptococcal infection—toxin producing, Kawasaki disease or Stevens–Johnson syndrome.
b. Examine the oral mucosa, lips and genitalia for signs of ulceration. The skin should be examined for erythema multiforme rash or macular rash, and the tonsils for signs of streptococcal sore throat. If Kawasaki disease is considered, one should look for cervical lymphadenopathy, conjunctivitis, fever, arthropathy and evidence of coronary artery aneurysms.

124.
a. Strangulation mark.
b. Protect the neck during airway opening procedures.

125.
a. • Haemolytic disease, haemoglobinopathies or thalassaemia
  • Infections—bacterial, viral or protozoan
  • Infiltration, e.g. Gaucher, Niemann–Pick
  • Neoplasms, leukaemia, Hodgkin's disease, neuroblastoma, nephroblastoma

- Macronodular cirrhosis
- Hepatic tumour
- Congestive, e.g. hepatic vein obstruction.

126.
a. Peripheral ischaemia after insertion of an umbilical arterial catheter.
b. The umbilical arterial catheter must be removed. Failure to do so may result in necrosis and gangrene of the peripheries.

127.
a. Erythema multiforme—vesiculobullous lesions that develop into target lesions. Involvement of mucous membranes occurs in Stevens–Johnson syndrome.
b. Causes include:
  - infection with viruses, such as herpes hominis, Coxsackie and echovirus, or bacteria including streptococcal infections and mycoplasma
  - drugs, e.g. penicillins, sulphonamides, barbiturates
  - collagen disorders
  - vaccines.
  Frequently, no cause can be found.
c. Treatment should be directed towards any identifiable cause. In addition, local and symptomatic therapy should be offered. Denuded skin areas can be cleansed with antiseptics, and topical anaesthetics may provide relief from pain. Patients may experience rapid relief following systemic corticosteroid therapy.

128.
a. Erysipelas—cellulitis with erythema, induration and well demarcated borders.
b. *Streptococcus pyogenes*—Lancefield group A β-haemolytic streptococcus.
c. Subcutaneous abscesses and bacteraemia which may result in metastatic foci.
d. Intravenous antibiotics, including penicillin and analgesia.

129.
a. Varicella zoster (shingles) involving dermatome T5.
b. Secondary bacterial infection and keratitis if the lesions involve the trigeminal nerve distribution. Postherpetic neuralgia is very rare in children.
c. Topical applications, e.g. calamine lotion. Acyclovir speeds the healing of lesions and may decrease pain.

130.
a. Target cells, Howell—Jolly bodies (blue-staining nuclear remnants of the red blood cells) and crenated red blood cells.
b. Hyposplenism. Splenectomy may be performed in chronic idiopathic thrombocytopenia and hereditary spherocytosis. Hyposplenism may also be secondary to congenital asplenia or sickle cell disease.

c. There is an increased risk of pyogenic infections including pneumonia, septicaemia and meningitis caused by pneumococcus and other polysaccharide encapsulated organisms (e.g. *Haemophilus influenzae* type B). *Haemophilus influenzae* type B vaccine should be given in infancy, and pneumococcal vaccine at 2 years of age or prior to splenectomy. Prophylactic antibiotics, usually penicillin, are recommended at least until adult life.

131.
a. This is a sagittal view of the pelvis. There is a well-rounded mass in the pelvis, superior to the bladder and uterus. It is heterogenous in appearance with a capsule.
b. The position would be consistent with a tumour arising from the ovary or uterus. At laparotomy, the mass was found to be a benign dermoid tumour.

132.
a. Lymphoedema of the feet.
b. Turner syndrome.
c. Karyotyping should be performed to look for Turner syndrome. The commonest karyotype in this condition is 45XO but many cases are mosaics. Eighty per cent of the lost chromosome are paternal in origin.
d. Low birth weight, short stature, webbing of the neck, shield chest, low hairline, cubitus valgus, coarctation of the aorta and bicuspid aortic valve, hypertension, horseshoe kidneys and streak ovaries. Children often have short stature and a lack of pubertal development.

133.
a. Facial hypoplasia with a depressed bridge of the nose and protrusion of the eyes. This would fit with craniofacial dysostosis (Crouzon disease), a condition characterised by craniosynostosis, beak-shaped nose, hypoplastic maxilla, protruding lower lip, exophthalmos and strabismus. Other conditions which feature craniosynostosis include Apert syndrome and Carpenter syndrome.
b. Surgical correction to bring forward the facial bones can be performed. Patients frequently require counselling to cope with the gross facial disharmony. Craniectomy along the prematurely fused suture may be indicated in the presence of craniosynostosis. This child has had several surgical procedures.

134.
a. Dehydration. The photographs demonstrate the loss of skin turgor.
b. The clinical assessment of dehydration is shown in the following table:

Clinical sign	5% dehydration (mild)	5–10% dehydration (moderate)	10% dehydration (severe)
Tachycardia	+	+ +	+ + +
Hypotension	−	−	+
Dry mouth	±	+	+
Thirst	+	±	−
Impaired skin turgor	−	±	+
Sunken eyes	−	+	+
Restless/apathy	−	+	+ +

The child should be weighed, and if a recent weight is known, this will give a more accurate assessment of the severity of the dehydration.

c. Children who are 10% or more dehydrated require careful resuscitation with intravenous fluids and monitoring of serum electrolytes. Milder forms of dehydration should be managed with oral rehydration solution for 24 hours before reintroducing foods. However, in the presence of profuse vomiting, intravenous therapy may be required even in mild dehydration.

135.

a. Electroencephalography. This procedure is performed to find supportive evidence of HIE. It can be used to differentiate seizures from events which may be difficult to distinguish clinically from fits. Severe background abnormalities such as excessive discontinuity, sudden burst of activity followed by abnormal suppression (burst suppression), or low voltage patterns are associated with a poor prognosis.

b. HIE is defined as abnormal neurological signs in the newborn period. Signs range from lethargy, mild irritability and hyperreflexia, to severe irritability, loss of primitive reflexes and seizures. Severe cases may be comatose, with absent or poor response to stimulation, areflexia, severe hypotonia and intractable seizures.

c. The infant will require monitoring of renal and liver function, and acid–base balance. Cranial ultrasound is useful to exclude other pathology and may show widespread echodensities in severe asphyxia. Magnetic resonance imaging (MRI) may show changes at a later stage. Lesions in the thalamic nuclei or dorsal striatum suggest a poor prognosis. Magnetic resonance spectroscopy may show signs of severe energy failure within 72 hours of the ischaemic event, which is of important prognostic significance, but this technique is not widely available.

136.
a. Impetigo—a superficial crusting skin infection with a yellow exudate. Caused by *Staphylococcus aureus* or β-haemolytic streptococcus.
b. This condition can spread and is contagious. If recurrent, it will be necessary to look for chronic nasal carriage of staphylococcus in the child and family.
c. Systemic antibiotics. Topical antibiotics may be used if there is only a minor infection.

137.
a. Epidermolysis bullosa—an inherited tendency to develop blisters within the skin with minimal trauma. Most affected infants develop lesions within the first few days after birth. The differential diagnosis includes other bullous lesions such as toxic epidermal necrolysis.
b. • *Simple epidermolysis bullosa*—non-scarring blisters mainly confined to the hands and feet. Inherited as autosomal dominant.
• *Junctional epidermolysis bullosa*—the rare but lethal variant involving the gastrointestinal tract. Inherited as autosomal recessive.
• *Dystrophic epidermolysis bullosa*—presents as scarring, pseudowebbing of the hands and feet, destruction of nails, and oesophageal strictures.
c. Careful nursing in the neonatal period with appropriate dressings. Patients may need periodic plastic procedures for release of digits. Iron therapy should be given to avoid anaemia, and intermittent antibiotic therapy may be required for skin infections. Parents should receive genetic counselling.

138.
a. Dilute urine. The urinanalysis dipstick shows a large amount of ketones and glucose.
b. Diabetic ketoacidosis.
c. Many young children with diabetic ketoacidosis are dehydrated and require resuscitation with intravenous saline followed by dextrose saline. Concurrently, intravenous short-acting insulin is administered at a dose determined by frequent blood glucose monitoring. The essentials of long-term management are diet, appropriate insulin and education about diabetes. Care is coordinated by a multidisciplinary team, including the paediatrician, family doctor, community nurse, dietician and school. Optimal diabetic control may reduce the long-term complications of diabetes.

139.
a. Nail clubbing.
b. Causes of clubbing, with or without cyanosis, are: **c**yanotic heart disease, **l**iver disease, **u**lcerative colitis or Crohn's disease, **b**ronchiectasis, e.g. cystic fibrosis, **in**fective endocarditis, **g**astrointestinal malabsorption.

140.
a. Head louse—pediculosis humanus capitis. Transmitted by direct contact. Leads to severe irritation, secondary infection and occipital lymph adenopathy.
b. Treatment is with malathion, permethrin or phenothrin. Carbaryl is no longer recommended. Most treatments need to be repeated 1 week later. After treatment, the nits must be combed out.
c. All regular contacts, including family members and contacts at school, must be treated. Sterilisation of clothing and combs is unnecessary.

141.
a. This X-ray shows a ground glass appearance to both lung fields, an air bronchogram and loss of the heart borders. Note the endotracheal tube.
b. This appearance is seen in hyaline membrane disease and group B haemolytic streptococcal pneumonia.
c. Air leak is common in neonates with hyaline membrane disease. X-ray may demonstrate pulmonary interstitial emphysema, pneumothorax, pneumomediastinum or pneumopericardium. In low birth weight infants, right upper lobe collapse from a poorly positioned endotracheal tube is common.

142.
a. Macroglossia—a large tongue.
b. This is seen in hypothyroidism and Beckwith–Wiedemann syndrome. Infants with Down syndrome have a similar appearance secondary to a small oropharynx. At a later age, macroglossia is a feature of mucopolysaccharidosis.

143.
a. Proptosis or exophthalmos—protrusion of the eye.
b. In this case, the cause of proptosis was an intracranial tumour. Other causes to consider include:
   • hyperthyroidism
   • shallowness of the orbits due to craniofacial malformations
   • increased tissue mass within the orbit, e.g. neoplastic and inflammatory conditions, especially neuroblastoma.
c. Ocular complications include exposure keratopathy, ocular motor disturbance and optic atrophy. Complications may arise from the underlying aetiology.
d. Urgent computed tomography or magnetic resonance imaging of the skull and orbit should be performed. Thyroid function tests should also be undertaken.

144.
a. Lesch–Nyhan syndrome. This photograph shows self-mutilation of the lips.
b. Delayed motor development, extrapyramidal choreoathetoid movements, hyperreflexia, spasticity, self-mutilation with lip and finger biting, and tophi.
c. Deficiency of hypoxanthine guanine phosphoribosyl transferase activity leading to accumulation of uric acid.
d. This is an X-linked condition.

145.
a. Group A streptococcal perianal cellulitis.
b. Anal swab for microbiological culture. Treat with a 10 day course of antibiotics; penicillin is the antibiotic of choice.
c. This condition has been confused with sexual abuse, which should of course be considered if there is supportive evidence. Other possible diagnoses to consider include anal fissure and perianal Crohn's disease.

146.
a. Atopic eczema—erythematous itchy rash typically involving the antecubital, popliteal fossa, and wrists.
b. Treatment includes emollient therapy, soap substitutes, topical steroids, oral anti-histamines, the use of cotton clothing and avoiding precipitants. Superadded infections should be treated early.
c. Uncertain but anecdotally up to one third of patients with eczema may improve on a milk and egg free diet.

147.
a. Massive tonsillar hypertrophy.
b. Airway obstruction, apnoea, difficulty in swallowing, post-streptococcal complications, e.g. peritonsillar abscess, suppurative cervical adenitis and otitis media.
c. Obstuctive sleep apnoea, frequent and severe tonsillitis not responding to appropriate antibiotics, failure to thrive and quinsy.

148.
a. Umbilical granuloma. The differential diagnosis is an umbilical polyp with persistence of the omphalomesenteric duct or urachus, which may discharge with faecal material or urine.
b. Umbilical granuloma are treated by cauterisation with silver nitrate. Care should be taken when applying silver nitrate to the granuloma to avoid staining the surrounding skin by the use of topical paraffin. Umbilical polyps need surgical excision with the omphalomesenteric or urachal remnant.

149.
a. Eczema herpeticum (superadded herpes simplex infection). Children with atopic eczema exhibit an abnormal response to herpes simplex which leads to dissemination of lesions with associated toxaemia.

b. The child should be admitted to hospital. Bacterial infection should be excluded and intravenous acyclovir commenced. Eczema therapy should be continued; oral antipruritic agents may be beneficial.

150.
a. Oral candidiasis with ulceration of the upper lip.
b. A swab should be taken for microscopy and culture.
c. Treatment is with an oral antifungal, e.g. nystatin and miconazole, and by regular mouth care whilst immunocompromised.

151.
a. Intrauterine growth retardation—the child is small for its gestational age.
b. Placental insufficiency, pre-eclampsia, maternal smoking, intrauterine infection, chromosomal abnormality or maternal renal disease.
c. Hypoglycaemia, polycythaemia, hypothermia and problems related to the aetiology of the intrauterine growth retardation. There is associated growth failure.

152.
a. Pityriasis rosea—widespread symmetrical rash on trunk and proximal limbs; oval $<$1 cm, pink macules which are covered by fine scales. Lesions may be arranged in a Christmas tree configuration along the cutaneous cleavage lines. The lesions may be preceded by a single dark red *herald patch*.
b. Treatment is usually unnecessary. Bland emollient will usually suffice, although topical corticosteroids are occasionally needed if there is severe pruritis.

153.
a. Sacrococcygeal teratoma.
b. They are often diagnosed antenatally by ultrasound. Lateral X-ray of the abdomen may show anterior displacement of the rectum, and a chest X-ray should be performed to identify pulmonary metastases. Further imaging with ultrasound or computed tomography may clarify the extent of the lesion. Serum alpha feto protein and chorionic gonadotrophin levels are often raised.
c. Only 10% of these tumours are malignant. They are more likely to be malignant if they can be palpated abdominally. If the teratoma is completely resected, the prognosis is excellent. Levels of alpha feto protein can be used to evaluate the effectiveness of surgery.

154.
a. Exomphalos—an abdominal wall defect covered by a sac of peritoneum, or hernia of the abdominal contents into the umbilical cord. This differs from gastroschisis where there is an intestinal herniation through an anterior wall defect

without peritoneal covering, usually to the right of the umbilicus.

b. Over 50% are associated with abnormalities of cardiovascular, genitourinary or gastrointestinal systems. There is an increased incidence in Beckwith–Wiedemann syndrome and Edward syndrome.

c. Surgical closure should be performed shortly after birth. During the procedure, the bowel should be closely inspected for atresias or stenoses. If the defect is large, it may be necessary to enclose the contents in an artificial membrane and slowly return the contents of the sac into the abdominal cavity over a period of days or weeks.

155.
a. Torn frenulum.
b. This can be caused by aggressively forcing a teat into a baby's mouth, and the clinician should suspect non-accidental injury.

156.
a. Anal atresia.
b. Urinary tract and vertebral abnormalities, perineal fistulae, rectovesical fistulae and other atresias, e.g. tracheo-oesophageal fistula.
c. Identify level of atresia—high lesions above the levator ani or low lesions, e.g. imperforate anus. High lesions require a preliminary colostomy followed by surgical repair and anorectoplasty, and are more lilely to be accompanied by urinary tract fistulae. Low lesions may just be a flap over the anus which can be incised.

157.
a. Swelling of the lips, angular cheilitis and perioral erythema. The diagnosis is Crohn's disease or orofacial granulomatosis. The two conditions are histologically identical, but the latter has no overt gastrointestinal manifestations of Crohn's disease. Orofacial granulomatosis may be related to food intolerance.
b. Crohn's disease in childhood is difficult to treat. Patients frequently require either corticosteroids or an elemental or polymeric diet to induce remission. The risk of relapse may be reduced with 5-aminosalicylate acid (5-ASA) therapy. Immunomodulator therapy such as azathioprine or cyclosporin can be used as steroid sparing agents. Up to 50% of children will require surgery within 15 years. Orofacial granulomatosis may resolve by avoiding aggravating foods.

158.
a. There is a large area of loss of brain tissue and cerebral atrophy on the left side. There is moderate ventricular dilatation, more on the left than on the right. There is a slightly widened interhemispheric fissure.

b. Left parietal lobe infarct.

c. The neonatal convulsions and abnormal neurological signs which may be present in the neonatal period after hypoxic ischaemic encephalopathy usually subside in the first few days or weeks after birth. A right hemiparesis or hemiplegia is likely and is usually clinically detected by the end of the first year of life. There is a risk of epilepsy, but intellectual development is usually normal in the absence of generalised cerebral atrophy.

159.

a. This photograph demonstrates petechial haemorrhages. The presence of low birth weight together with hepatosplenomegaly suggests a congenital viral infection, most commonly cytomegalovirus (CMV) or rubella. Congenital toxoplasmosis is more common in Europe than in Britain and, although uncommon, may present with petechiae and hepatosplenomegaly. Other causes of neonatal thrombocytopenia leading to petechiae include transplacental passage of antiplatelet antibodies against platelet-specific antigens (neonatal alloimmune thrombocytopenia), neonatal bacterial septicaemia, disseminated intravascular coagulation, maternal pre-eclampsia and other hypertensive disorders and maternal conditions such as systemic lupus erythematosus.

b. Features of congenital rubella include intrauterine growth retardation, microcephaly, microphthalmia, cataracts, glaucoma, chorioretinitis, hepatosplenomegaly and neonatal jaundice. There is an increased risk of patent ductus arteriosus, anaemia and leucopenia. X-ray of long bones may demonstrate metaphyseal translucencies ('celery stalk' femur). The majority of affected children will have sensorineural deafness, but some infants may be asymptomatic. Ninety per cent of infants with congenital CMV are asymptomatic in the neonatal period and of normal birth weight, but those with multisystem disease may present with petechiae, hepatosplenomegaly, low birth weight and microcephaly.

c. The rubella virus and CMV can usually be isolated from urine. Serum should be taken to measure rubella and CMV-specific IgM. Eyes should be examined for chorioretinitis, and intracranial imaging may demonstrate periventricular calcification in congenital CMV.

160.

a. Henoch–Schönlein purpura—a multi-organ disease most frequently affecting the skin, joints and gastrointestinal tract. It is associated with a small vessel vasculitis.

b. • Cutaneous: purpuric rash
   • Abdominal: vomiting, melaena, intussusception and bowel perforation

- Arthopathy: usually involving the large joints
- Renal: haematuria, proteinuria, glomerulonephritis
- Neurological: cerebral vasculitis, intracranial haemorrhage, seizures.

c. In mild cases, it is sufficient to treat symptomatically and monitor for serious complications of the disease. Steroid therapy is indicated for severe abdominal pain, testicular pain, pulmonary haemorrhage or severe renal involvement.

161.
a. Bilateral ptosis, which is more marked on the left.
b. Juvenile onset of myasthenia gravis.
c. Demonstration of progressive weakness after repetitive movement, presence of acetylcholine receptor antibody in the blood, and response to anticholinesterase drugs, e.g. endrophonium test. Thymoma should be excluded.
d. Treatment is with pyridostigmine or neostigmine. Beware of toxicity, e.g. colic, diarrhoea, salivation, bradycardia, respiratory difficulty. One should avoid drugs that exacerbate symptoms and admit the patient to hospital during myasthenic crises. Other therapies include steroids (with potassium supplements), gammaglobulin in the severely ill, and thymectomy.

162.
a. Kawasaki disease.
b. Fever persisting for 5 days plus four of the following five clinical signs:
  - erythema and swelling of the palms and soles progressing to desquamation as shown in the photograph
  - polymorphous rash
  - bilateral conjunctival congestion
  - reddening and cracking of lips, with strawberry tongue
  - marked cervical lymphadenopathy.
  Thrombocytosis commonly occurs in the second week of the illness.
c. Coronary artery aneurysms and thrombosis are the most serious complications and are more common in children under the age of 1 year. Other less common complications include uveitis, aseptic meningitis and arthritis.
d. The diagnosis is often difficult to make in the early stages. Intravenous immunoglobulin and aspirin therapy reduce the complication rate if given early. Steroids have not been shown to affect the prognosis.

163.
a. Cutaneous larva migrans (creeping eruption). This is caused by a filariform larva of the dog or cat hookworm penetrating the skin. An itchy papule develops and the tract of the larva progresses at 1–2 mm/day. Healing occurs by crusting. In this

case, the child had spent her vacation in the West Indies playing with an infected local dog.

b. Treatment is with local topical or oral thiabendazole.

164.
a. Left facial nerve palsy (cranial nerve VII).
b. In this age group, the lesion is usually from pressure over the facial nerve in utero during labour. Most facial nerve palsies occur after normal vaginal delivery, but there is an increased incidence after forceps extraction. One should examine for other cranial nerve injuries, e.g. abducens nerve (cranial nerve VI). Rarely, the lesion may be due to nuclear agenesis of the facial nerve.
c. Ninety per cent recover fully within the first week of life. If the facial nerve palsy persists, surgery can be performed at a later age by introducing the functioning VIIth nerve motor fibres from the unparalysed side of the face.

165.
a. Ampicillin-induced rash with infectious mononucleosis.
b. Epstein–Barr virus.
c. Swelling of tonsils causing respiratory obstruction, splenic rupture, convulsions, ataxia, Guillain–Barré, myocarditis, interstitial pneumonia and haemolytic anaemia.

166.
a. This photograph shows short deformed limbs due to intrauterine fractures. This occurs in osteogenesis imperfecta. This appearance can be confused with chondroplasia (short-limbed dwarfism), but the diagnosis can be established radiographically.
b. The prognosis for osteogenesis imperfecta depends on the type. Severely affected infants are often stillborn or die in early infancy. Milder forms of osteogenesis imperfecta have less severe bone fragility and some have blue sclerae. Children who survive beyond infancy may have serious orthopaedic deformity and deafness. Children with achondroplasia have delayed early motor development and severe short stature but usually have normal intellectual ability.

167.
a. This photograph shows a depressed skull fracture involving the frontal bone which was related to birth trauma.
b. Imaging with magnetic resonance imaging or computed tomography will be indicated to exclude an associated subdural haemorrhage or cerebral contusion.

168.
a. Truncal obesity, interscapular fat pad, striae, gynaecomastia and facial plethora.
b. Cushing's syndrome.
c. Exogenous corticosteroids, pituitary adenoma, adrenal adenoma or carcinoma, or ectopic ACTH production.

d. Blood sampling for midnight cortisol, low- and high-dose dexamethasone suppression test, adrenal and pituitary imaging.

169.
a. Ranula—a superficial mucous retention cyst in the anterior part of the floor of the mouth, displacing the tongue due to partial obstruction of the submandibular or sublingual duct.
b. They usually subside spontaneously, but occasionally need marsupialisation if persistent.

170.
a. Periventricular calcification, dilated ventricles and cerebral atrophy.
b. Congenital cytomegalovirus (CMV) or toxoplasmosis infection. Calcification in CMV is more periventricular and less diffuse than in toxoplasmosis.
c. CMV infection is common in pregnancy, and up to 1% of normal healthy infants may excrete the virus in the urine. Some of these children are found to be deaf and have learning difficulties. A small number of newborn babies are symptomatic and may demonstrate intrauterine growth retardation, microcephaly, chorioretinitis, intracranial calcification, jaundice, mild hepatitis, hepatomegaly, haemolytic anaemia and thrombocytopenia.

   Toxoplasma is more common on the European continent than in the UK. Most infants are asymptomatic in the newborn period. Symptomatic babies may demonstrate some of the following features: hydrocephaly, microcephaly, chorioretinitis, cerebral calcifications, fits, developmental delay, thrombocytopenia, hepatosplenomegaly, jaundice.

171.
a. Gangrenous bowel with gastrointestinal perforation secondary to necrotising enterocolitis (NEC).
b. Abdominal distension, bile-stained aspirate, vomiting and bloody mucous stools. The infant may have recurrent apnoea, and if associated with peritonitis, the patient may be extremely unwell with hypotension and poor peripheral perfusion.
c. Risk factors include preterm birth, low birth weight, intrauterine growth retardation, birth asphyxia, artificial feeds, polycythaemia, exchange transfusion and cannulation of the umbilical vessels. Term infants may occasionally develop NEC.
d. Treatment is medical, with cessation of feeds, passage of large nasogastric tube, correction of shock and acidosis, ventilation, total parenteral nutrition and broad-spectrum antibiotics. Peritoneal drainage may be indicated. Surgery may be

considered if there is gross abdominal distension or perforation.

e. Poor prognostic features are extensive disease, persistent acidosis, renal failure, birth weight <1000 g, and failure to respond to conservative treatment.

172.
a. Noonan syndrome.
b. Short stature, webbing of neck, cubitus valgus, hypertelorism, epicanthic folds, ptosis, antimongoloid palpebral slant, variable developmental delay, cryptorchidism, pubertal delay, cardiac defects, e.g. dysplastic pulmonary valve, pulmonary stenosis, left ventricular hypertrophy or secundum atrial septal defect, feeding difficulties.
c. Approximately half are sporadic, but autosomal dominant inheritance with variable expression is well established.

173.
a. Hydrocephalus with enlarged head, 'setting sun' sign of the eyes and a convergent squint.
b. Causes include:
- posthaemorrhagic hydrocephalus following intraventricular haemorrhage
- aqueduct stenosis
- post-meningitis
- spina bifida.

174.
a. Anogenital warts (condyloma acuminata).
b. The clinician should suspect sexual abuse in children with anogenital warts, although those under 2 years of age are less likely to have been abused and may have been exposed to human papillomavirus before or at the time of delivery.
c. The possibility of child sexual abuse must be considered. A multidisciplinary approach with interagency colaboration between a paediatrician, social worker and child protection team is necessary to assess the child and social circumstances. Local guidelines should be followed. Tests for other sexually transmitted diseases should be performed, and if positive this confirms the diagnosis of sexual abuse. The family and index case must be interviewed and counselled appropriately.

175.
a. Single palmar crease.
b. This is a normal finding in 10–15% of briths. It is more often associated with Down syndrome and other trisomies.
c. Down syndrome is associated with clinodactyly of the 5th digit. In infants with trisomy 18, the hand is often clenched, with hypoplastic nails and a distal crease. The 5th finger may be absent. Postaxial polydactyly, hyperconvex fingernails and clenched hands are seen in trisomy 13.

176.
a. Neonatal jaundice.
b. Jaundice *with the first 24 hours of age* suggests acute haemolysis, most commonly secondary to rhesus or ABO incompatibility, or bacterial sepsis.
c. Serial determination of the total bilirubin is required in all jaundiced infants. The blood group of the infant and mother should be obtained to identify ABO or rhesus incompatibility. A positive Coomb's test in the infant confirms the presence of antibodies against the red cells. Serial haemoglobin or packed cell volume will determine if there is ongoing haemolysis, and blood film should be performed to look for abnormal cells, e.g. spherocytes. A full infection screen may be indicated if the infant is unwell.
d. The infant may require phototherapy and fluid replacement if dehydrated. Antibiotics should be administered if infection is suspected. If the bilirubin is rising rapidly or the infant is preterm or sick, exchange transfusion may be required.

177.
a. Purpura fulminans.
b. The most likely cause is meningococcal septicaemia. It can also occur after varicella zoster infection or pneumococcal disease.
c. The child may require resuscitation and transfer to intensive care for ventilation, colloid infusion, inotrope therapy for myocardial dysfunction, correction of electrolyte disturbance and acidosis, and treatment of the coagulopathy. High-dose intravenous third-generation cephalosporin or penicillin should be administered early, and acyclovir given if associated with chickenpox.

178.
a. Pubertal delay and wasting.
b. The combination of pubertal delay and wasting is a feature of inflammatory bowel disease, especially Crohn's disease, poor nutrition, anorexia nervosa, intestinal malabsorption and chronic illnesses such as cystic fibrosis or chronic renal failure.
c. A detailed history should be taken with particular reference to diet, and thorough examination should be performed. A bone age assessment (X-ray of wrist) should be performed, and measurement of ESR or C-reactive protein, full blood count and routine biochemistry carried out. Consider colonoscopy and barium meal and follow-through to investigate for inflammatory bowel disease. Endocrine investigations may be indicated to assess the hypothalamic pituitary axis and thyroid function.

Index